# Partial to Total Nasal Reconstruction

*Editor*

SAMUEL L. OYER

# FACIAL PLASTIC SURGERY CLINICS OF NORTH AMERICA

www.facialplastic.theclinics.com

*Consulting Editor*
ANTHONY P. SCLAFANI

May 2024 • Volume 32 • Number 2

**ELSEVIER**

1600 John F. Kennedy Boulevard • Suite 1800 • Philadelphia, Pennsylvania, 19103-2899

http://www.theclinics.com

**FACIAL PLASTIC SURGERY CLINICS OF NORTH AMERICA Volume 32, Number 2**
**May 2024 ISSN 1064-7406, ISBN-13: 978-0-443-12885-1**

Editor: Stacy Eastman
Developmental Editor: Shivank Joshi

*Facial Plastic Surgery Clinics of North America* (ISSN 1064-7406) is published quarterly by Elsevier Inc., 360 Park Avenue South, New York, NY 10010-1710. Months of issue are February, May, August, and November. Business and Editorial Offices: 1600 John F. Kennedy Blvd., Suite 1800, Philadelphia, PA 19103-2899. Periodicals postage paid at New York, NY, and additional mailing offices. Subscription prices are $432.00 per year (US individuals), $487.00 per year (Canadian individuals), $579.00 per year (foreign individuals), $100.00 per year (US students), $100.00 per year (Canadian students), and $255.00 per year (foreign students). For institutional access pricing please contact Customer Service via the contact information below. Foreign air speed delivery is included in all *Clinics* subscription prices. All prices are subject to change without notice. POSTMASTER: Send address changes to *Facial Plastic Surgery Clinics*, Elsevier Health Sciences Division, Subscription Customer Service, 3251 Riverport Lane, Maryland Heights, MO 63043. **Customer service: 1-800-654-2452 (US and Canada); 1-314-447-8871 (outside US and Canada); Fax: 314-447-8029; E-mail: journalscustomerservice-usa@elsevier.com (for print support); journalsonline-support-usa@elsevier.com (for online support).**

*Reprints.* For copies of 100 or more of articles in this publication, please contact the Commercial Reprints Department, Elsevier Inc., 360 Park Avenue South, New York, NY 10010-1710. Tel.: 212-633-3874; Fax: 212-633-3820; E-mail: reprints@elsevier.com.

*Facial Plastic Surgery Clinics of North America* is covered in *MEDLINE/PubMed* (*Index Medicus*).

# Contributors

## CONSULTING EDITOR

**ANTHONY P. SCLAFANI, MD, MBA, FACS**
Director of Facial Plastic Surgery, Professor of
Otolaryngology- Head & Neck Surgery, Weill
Cornell Medical College, New York, New York

## EDITOR

**SAMUEL L. OYER, MD**
Associate Professor, Facial Plastic and
Reconstructive Surgery, Department of
Otolaryngology–Head and Neck Surgery,
University of Virginia, Charlottesville, Virginia

## AUTHORS

**KHASHAYAR ARIANPOUR, MD**
ENT-otolaryngologist, Head and Neck
Institute, Cleveland Clinic, Cleveland, Ohio

**SCOTT BEVANS, MD**
Associate Professor, Uniformed Services
University, Bethesda, Maryland;
Otolaryngologists, Department of
Otolaryngology, Tripler Army Medical Center,
Honolulu, Hawaii

**SYDNEY C. BUTTS, MD**
Interim Chair and Associate Professor, Chief of
Facial Plastic and Reconstructive Surgery,
Department of Otolaryngology, SUNY
Downstate Health Sciences University,
Brooklyn, New York

**PATRICK J. BYRNE, MD, MBA**
Chief, Head and Neck Institute, Cleveland
Clinic, Cleveland, Ohio

**MICHAELA CALHOUN, MS, CCA**
Certified Anaplastologist, Owner and Clinical
Director, Medical Art Resources, Inc and
Prosthetics at Graphica Medica, Milwaukee,
Wisconsin

**JOSEPH MADISON CLARK, MD, FACS**
Chair and W. Paul Biggers Distinguished
Professor, Division of Facial Plastic and
Reconstructive Surgery, University of
North Carolina, Chapel Hill, North
Carolina

**BETSY K. DAVIS, DMD, MS**
Maxillofacial Prosthodontist, Head and Neck
Specialists-Charleston, National Director of
Maxillofacial Prosthodontics and Dental
Oncology, HCA Healthcare and Sarah
Cannon Cancer Institute, Nashville,
Tennessee

**VIRGINIA E. DRAKE, MD**
Assistant Professor, Division of Facial Plastic
and Reconstructive Surgery, Department of
Otolaryngology–Head and Neck Surgery,
University of North Carolina, Chapel Hill, North
Carolina

**JOHN L. FRODEL Jr, MD**
Attending Physician, Guthrie Medical Group,
Guthrie Ithaca City Harbor, Otolaryngology,
Facial Plastic Surgery, Ithaca, New York

**SHEKHAR K. GADKAREE, MD**
Assistant Professor, Division of Facial Plastic and Reconstructive Surgery, Department of Otolaryngology–Head and Neck Surgery, University of Miami Miller School of Medicine, Miami, Florida

**ALEXANDER E. GRAF, MD**
Resident Physician, Department of Otolaryngology, SUNY Downstate Health Sciences University, Brooklyn, New York

**BRITTANY E. HOWARD, MD**
Division Chair and Assistant Professor, Division of Facial Plastic and Reconstructive Surgery, Mayo Clinic Arizona, Phoenix, Arizona

**HANNAH JACOBS-EL, MPH**
Medical Student, Department of Otolaryngology–Head and Neck Surgery, University of Virginia, Charlottesville, Virginia

**LEE KAPLOWITZ, MD**
Attending Surgeon, Division of Otolaryngology, Department of Surgery, Maimonides Medical Center, Brooklyn, New York

**LESLIE R. KIM, MD**
Clinical Associate Professor, Department of Otolaryngology–Head and Neck Surgery, Ohio State Eye and Ear Institute, Columbus, Ohio State University Wexner Medical Center, Ohio

**CORIN M. KINKHABWALA, MD**
Resident Surgeon, Department of Otolaryngology Head and Neck Surgery, Medical University of South Carolina, Charleston, South Carolina

**HANNAH N. KUHAR, MD**
Resident Physician, Department of Otolaryngology–Head and Neck Surgery, Ohio State Eye and Ear Institute, Columbus, Ohio State University Wexner Medical Center, Ohio

**JESSYKA G. LIGHTHALL, MD**
Associate Professor, Division of Facial Plastic and Reconstructive Surgery, Department of Otolaryngology–Head and Neck Surgery, Penn State College of Medicine, Hershey, Pennsylvania

**JEFFREY MELLA, MD**
Chief Resident, Department of Otolaryngology–Head and Neck Surgery, University of Virginia, Charlottesville, Virginia

**JEFFREY S. MOYER, MD**
Professor, Division of Facial Plastic and Reconstructive Surgery, Department of Otolaryngology–Head and Neck Surgery, University of Michigan, Ann Arbor, Michigan

**RYAN NESEMEIER, MD**
Physician, Department of Otolaryngology–Head and Neck Surgery, Ohio State Eye and Ear Institute, Ohio State University Wexner Medical Center, Columbus, Ohio

**SAMUEL L. OYER, MD**
Associate Professor, Facial Plastic and Reconstructive Surgery, Department of Otolaryngology–Head and Neck Surgery, University of Virginia, Charlottesville, Virginia

**STEPHEN S. PARK, MD**
Professor & Chair, Department of Otolaryngology–Head and Neck Surgery, University of Virginia, Charlottesville, Virginia

**KRISHNA G. PATEL, MD, PhD**
Professor and Division Chief of Facial Plastic and Reconstructive Surgery, Department of Otolaryngology–Head and Neck Surgery, Medical University of South Carolina, Charleston, South Carolina

**SAMIP PATEL, MD, FACS**
Associate Professor, Division of Head and Neck Surgery, Mayo Clinic Florida, Jacksonville, Florida

**MICHELLE K. RUSE, DDS, MDS**
Maxillofacial Prosthodontist, Head and Neck Specialists-Charleston, HCA Healthcare and Sarah Cannon Cancer Institute, Nashville, Tennessee

**HEATHER K. SCHOPPER, MD**
Facial Plastic and Reconstructive Surgery Fellow, Division of Facial Plastic and Reconstructive Surgery, Department of Otolaryngology–Head and Neck Surgery, Penn State College of Medicine, Hershey, Pennsylvania

**TAHA Z. SHIPCHANDLER, MD**
Professor, Division Chief of Facial Plastic and Reconstructive Surgery, Department of Otolaryngology—Head and Neck Surgery, Indiana University School of Medicine

**WILLIAM W. SHOCKLEY, MD, FACS**
Emeritus Professor, Division of Facial Plastic and Reconstructive Surgery, University of North Carolina, Chapel Hill, North Carolina

**STEPHEN P. SMITH Jr, MD**
Surgeon, Smith Facial Plastics, Columbus Ohio, Gahanna, Ohio

**JIN SOO SONG, MD**
Smith Facial Plastics, Columbus Ohio, Gahanna, Ohio

**CHAZ L. STUCKEN, MD**
Clinical associate professor, Department of Otolaryngology–Head and Neck Surgery, University of Michigan, Ann Arbor, Michigan

**BETSY SZETO, MD, MPH**
Chief Resident, Department of Otolaryngology–Head and Neck Surgery, University of Virginia, Charlottesville, Virginia

**DOMINIC VERNON, MD**
Assistant Professor, Department of Otolaryngology-Head & Neck Surgery, Indiana University School of Medicine, Avon, Indiana

# Contents

> Owing to the complex, multilayered anatomy of the nose in the central face, major nasal reconstruction can pose a significant challenge for reconstructive surgeons. It is the responsibility of reconstructive surgeons to have an understanding of the most common cutaneous malignancies and excisional techniques that may lead to complex nasal defects. The purpose of this article is to discuss these malignancies, excisional techniques, and impacts of radiation on tissue that has implications for reconstructive surgeons.

> This article reviews special considerations in complex nasal defects including treatment of adjacent subunit defects, timing of repair with radiation, reconstruction in patients with prior repairs or recurrent disease, and the role of prosthetics. The role of technological advances including virtual surgical planning, 3 dimensional printing, biocompatible materials, and tissue engineering is discussed.

> In this review, the paramedian forehead flap indications and uses are reviewed, specifically examining clinical situations where patient selection is important. In these settings, a preoperative discussion with a patient regarding surgical expectations and goals in the setting of their defect is paramount. The authors review the literature regarding the psychosocial aspects of major nasal reconstruction and review preoperative discussion points that are key to a well-informed patient and improved patient satisfaction through the nasal reconstructive process.

> Defects over 2.0 to 2.5 cm may often require repair with a multistaged forehead flap. However, in some such defects, other options may be available. In this article, the author will review some of these options.

and internal lining grafts, this flap remains the workhorse flap for resurfacing large nasal defects. Various nuances of this technique relating to defect and template preparation, flap design, flap elevation, flap inset, donor site closure, and pedicle division are discussed in this article. These nuances are the guiding principles for improved outcomes using a forehead flap for the reconstruction of large nasal defects.

Prosthetic nasal reconstruction provides a restorative option for patients with nasal defects, and these can be retained with a variety of methods including adhesives and implants. These prostheses can significantly improve appearance, self-esteem, and quality of life for patients and they restore many functions of the external nose. Traditional fabrication methods are often used by the skilled professionals who make these custom prostheses, but digital technology is improving the workflow for design and fabrication of silicone nasal prostheses. Nasal prosthetic reconstruction requires multidisciplinary coordination between surgeons, maxillofacial prosthodontists, anaplastologists, and other members of the healthcare team. Prosthetic treatment can be considered as an alternative to, or an addition to treatment with surgical reconstruction.

# FACIAL PLASTIC SURGERY CLINICS OF NORTH AMERICA

**THE CLINICS ARE AVAILABLE ONLINE!**
Access your subscription at:
www.theclinics.com

# Foreword
# Nasal Reconstruction

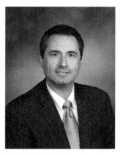

Anthony P. Sclafani, MD, MBA, FACS
*Consulting Editor*

*If I have seen further than others, it is by standing upon the shoulders of giants.*
— *Isaac Newton*

Nasal reconstruction, whether small or large, continues to be a challenge for facial plastic surgeons. Despite better patient awareness, skin surveillance, and micrographic excision, surgeons still are frequently faced with large and complex nasal defects. While the patient, prior to Mohs excision, is told to "hope for the best," the prudent surgeon must be "prepared for the worst." That preparation is critical to the surgical outcome and the patient's life.

Guest Editor, Samuel L. Oyer, MD, has assembled an outstanding group of authors who write about their experience dealing with these "worst-case scenarios"—truly challenging nasal defects. These authors approach reconstruction of significant nasal injuries from an anatomic perspective and share their experience with established and novel techniques of total nasal reconstruction.

We feel fortunate any time we can benefit from the wisdom of a single "giant" in the field, but *each* article in this issue of *Facial Plastic Surgery Clinics of North America* is authored by at least one "giant,"

collectively too numerous and personally too modest to list by name. These articles will help you better prepare for those "worst-case scenarios" that often seem to come without warning. The reader of this issue is invited to feast on the broad spectrum and richness of the knowledge and experience shared by these authors. I hope you enjoy this issue of *Facial Plastic Surgery Clinics of North America*!

*Scientists are not dependent on the ideas of a single man, but on the combined wisdom of thousands of men, all thinking of the same problem, and each doing his little bit to add to the great structure of knowledge which is gradually being erected.*
— *Ernest Rutherford*

Anthony P. Sclafani, MD, MBA, FACS
Director of Facial Plastic Surgery
Professor of Otolaryngology- Head & Neck Surgery
Weill Cornell Medical College
New York, NY 10021, USA

Facial Plast Surg Clin N Am 32 (2024) xiii
https://doi.org/10.1016/j.fsc.2024.02.002
1064-7406/24/© 2024 Published by Elsevier Inc.

facialplastic.theclinics.com

# Preface
# Major Nasal Reconstruction: Rising to the Challenge

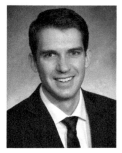

Samuel L. Oyer, MD
*Editor*

Even a small nasal defect presents a significant challenge for the reconstructive surgeon. The functional and aesthetic demands of an ideal reconstruction are tremendously high when aiming for a flawless reconstruction of the most central feature of the face. The complexity of this task increases exponentially for large nasal defects or those that involve structure and lining in addition to skin. Reconstruction of extensive subtotal or total nasal defects is a daunting endeavor often faced only a handful of times throughout a reconstructive surgeon's career.

Despite the complexity of the task, we have more knowledge and technology available today than at any point in the history of medicine. The standards to which we hold our nasal reconstructions have also increased substantially over time. No longer is the goal simply to "fill the defect" but rather to create an inconspicuous and normal-appearing nose with normal nasal function. Even among the most challenging nasal defects, this is where the reconstructive bar is set.

We owe our current reconstructive capabilities to numerous influential pioneers that have come before us; we truly stand on the shoulders of giants who were not content accepting the status quo of subpar reconstruction. From its roots in antiquity, the art of nasal reconstruction has progressed thanks to the relentless work by countless surgeons. Sir Charles Gillies leveraged his experience

treating traumatic wartime injuries to pioneer several novel surgical techniques and taught us the value of staging surgical steps to optimize success. Similarly, the collective works of Drs Fred Menick and Gary Burget truly redefined the way we look at a nose using the subunit principle and raised the bar in terms of reconstructive precision and outcomes. The complete list of surgeons who have added to our knowledge of nasal reconstruction is too long to enumerate here, but what is clear is that we could not offer patients the level of nasal reconstruction available today without an acknowledgment of the tremendous efforts of those who came before us.

What follows in this issue is the contemporary state of nasal reconstruction. The pearls and perils in these articles represent the collective experience of more than a dozen reconstructive surgeons with nearly 300 years of collective clinical experience. By collating this experience, I hope the reader will gain a solid foundation of the fundamentals of nasal reconstruction along with a respect for and recognition of potential complications that can derail a reconstruction. With this knowledge, some common pitfalls may be avoided, as it is always best to learn from others' mistakes without the need to repeat them all oneself. Building on these foundations, the reader will also explore cutting-edge techniques in nasal reconstruction, including prelamination of flaps,

Facial Plast Surg Clin N Am 32 (2024) xv–xvi
https://doi.org/10.1016/j.fsc.2024.01.001
1064-7406/24/© 2024 Published by Elsevier Inc.

**facialplastic.theclinics.com**

use of novel free flaps, and the application of technology to aid in the quest for perfect nasal reconstruction. Contemporary use of nasal prosthetics is also discussed to ensure the reconstructive surgeon is familiar with all possible treatment modalities of a nasal defect.

Our charge as reconstructive surgeons is to pursue the goal of near-perfect nasal reconstruction wholeheartedly. By applying the fundamental techniques established by our predecessors, critically analyzing and refining our own results, and collectively sharing our successes and failures, we can continue to raise the bar of nasal reconstruction. Together, we can work toward the ideal of a flawless and functional nose.

Samuel L. Oyer, MD
Facial Plastic and Reconstructive Surgery
Department of Otolaryngology–Head and Neck
Surgery
University of Virginia
PO Box 800173
Charlottesville, VA 22908, USA

*E-mail address:*
SLO5FA@uvahealth.org

# Implications of Malignancy, Radiation, and Timing of Major Nasal Reconstruction

Jin Soo Song, MD[a], Stephen P. Smith Jr, MD[a], Chaz L. Stucken, MD[b],*

## KEYWORDS

• Nasal reconstruction • Skin cancer • Mohs • Timing

## KEY POINTS

• Complex Nasal Anatomy: The central face's intricate, multilayered nasal anatomy presents a significant challenge for reconstructive surgeons during major nasal reconstruction.
• Surgeon's Responsibility: Reconstructive surgeons must be well-versed in common cutaneous malignancies and excisional techniques, as these can result in complex nasal defects.
• Discussion on Malignancies: This article aims to discuss various cutaneous malignancies commonly encountered, shedding light on their characteristics and implications for nasal reconstruction.
• Excisional Techniques: The article also delves into excisional techniques used in addressing these malignancies, providing insights for reconstructive surgeons in managing complex cases.
• Radiation's Impact: In addition, the article explores how radiation therapy affects tissues, offering valuable knowledge for surgeons dealing with postradiation reconstructive challenges.

## BACKGROUND

The incidence of cutaneous melanoma (CM) and nonmelanoma skin cancer (NMSC) is increasing both within the United States and on a global scale. Within the United States, this is represented by one in five Americans being diagnosed with skin cancer by age 70 years.[1] For NMSC, up to 95% are diagnosed in the head and neck (H&N) region due to ultraviolet light exposure.[2] Furthermore, more than 50% of individuals will develop a second primary NMSC within 5 years.[2] The incidence of CM has increased by 51.1% over 20 years in pediatric and young adult populations, with approximately 20% of CM occurring in the H&N.[3] Skin cancer places a substantial health and economic burden on health care systems. The overall treatment cost of skin cancers within the United States is estimated to be more than $8.1 billion annually.[4]

Treatment and reconstruction of these increasingly prevalent H&N cutaneous malignancies poses a challenging feat. The difficulty arises from the prominently visible location of the nose and its role in essential functions including smell and breathing. Therefore, optimizing reconstruction following a complete oncologic resection of these malignancies carries a heightened importance. As the nose acts as the center piece of the face, with nuanced three-dimensional contours and variability in skin composition, it is a particularly difficult area for reconstruction. This is corroborated by previous reports demonstrating skin cancer repair on the nose as an independent

[a] Smith Facial Plastics, Columbus Ohio, 725 Buckles Court North #210, Gahanna, OH 43230, USA; [b] Department of Otolaryngology – Head and Neck Surgery, University of Michigan, 1500 East Medical Center Drive, Ann Arbor, MI 48109, USA
* Corresponding author.
E-mail address: cstucken@med.umich.edu

Facial Plast Surg Clin N Am 32 (2024) 189–198
https://doi.org/10.1016/j.fsc.2023.12.001
1064-7406/24/© 2023 Elsevier Inc. All rights reserved.

predictive factor in patient's postoperative psychosocial distress.[5] Furthermore, the multilayered skin, cartilage and mucosal reconstruction of full thickness defects, requires a more complex reconstruction. Among the many considerations to optimize a nasal repair, the decision of timing of reconstruction is an area of contention. Herein, the authors discuss the variables implicated in determining the best timing for nasal reconstruction following skin cancer resection.

## RESECTION MODALITIES

The eradication of malignancy before reconstruction is of paramount importance to the reconstructive surgeon. The current clinical consensus on recommended surgical resection techniques for skin cancers predominantly consists of wide local excision (WLE), Mohs micrographic surgery (MMS), and staged excision.[6]

### Wide Local Excision

Within WLE, the surgical specimen is assessed via vertical bread-loaf sectioning, which examines only about 1% of the surgical margin (**Fig. 1**). Therefore, making a determination on margin clearance is considered a calculated decision rather than a true clearance.[6,7] When intraoperative frozen section analysis is performed, inaccuracies of margin status may arise from gross sampling errors by the surgeon, misinterpretation of the frozen section biopsy by the pathologist, or sampling error due to the technique of only analyzing a portion of the specimen.[8] Facial plastic and reconstructive surgeons should be aware of the risk of false-negative results for frozen section analysis of high-risk basal cell carcinoma (BCC) and SCC of the H&N, as one large retrospective analysis of these cases demonstrated frozen section false-negative rates of 28.7% and 27.5%, respectively.[8] When WLE is performed with postoperative margin assessment, healing by

secondary intention, linear repair, or skin grafting are acceptable options. Local flaps, extensive undermining, or tissue rearrangement should only be performed once clear margins are identified.

### Mohs Micrographic Surgery

MMS is generally considered a favorable technique for NMSC, as peripheral and deep tissue is prepared and examined by the Mohs surgeon from the flattened tissue for complete margin analysis (**Fig. 2**).[6] Because 100% of the margin face can be examined, margin control is more reliable than standard WLE for NMSC. The primary advantage of the Mohs technique is that facial plastic and reconstructive surgeons can perform local tissue rearrangement and reconstruction immediately rather than in a delayed fashion.

A prospective randomized trial compared MMS with WLE for primary and recurrent BCC. MMS versus WLE showed 10-year recurrence rates for primary BCC of 2.5 vs. 4.1% ($P = .397$) and recurrent BCC of 2.4 versus 12.1% ($P = .15$).[9] These findings occurred with an initial 3 mm resection margin for both treatment arms, which resulted in complete resection within two stages for 78% of MMS cases.[9] In addition, MMS offers the advantage of tissue sparing compared with WLE. A study of 30 patients with subcentimetric facial BCC treated with WLE and MMS incorporating 4 and 2 mm margins, respectively, yielded resultant median area of surgical defects of 116.6 mm$^2$ and 187.7 mm$^2$, respectively.[10] Likewise, a prospective study of 256 primary facial and scalp BCCs compared suspected defect surface area incorporating 5 mm surgical margins for WLE versus actual surface area following MMS. With a median tumor size of 71 mm$^2$, the median defect size following MMS versus expected WLE defect dimensions was 154 mm$^2$ and 298 mm$^2$, respectively, resulting in a 46.4% tissue sparing effect.[11] However, MMS remains a controversial

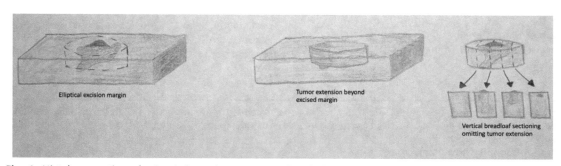

Elliptical excision margin

Tumor extension beyond excised margin

Vertical breadloaf sectioning omitting tumor extension

**Fig. 1.** Histology section obtained through conventional wide local excision. (Artwork performed by Emily Z. Stucken, MD.)

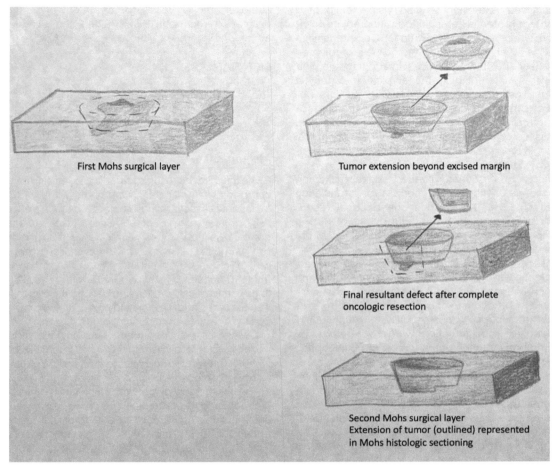

First Mohs surgical layer

Tumor extension beyond excised margin

Final resultant defect after complete oncologic resection

Second Mohs surgical layer
Extension of tumor (outlined) represented in Mohs histologic sectioning

**Fig. 2.** Histology section obtained through Mohs micrographic surgery. (Artwork performed by Emily Z. Stucken, MD.)

option for CM, and permanent section analysis remains the gold standard.[12]

Yet, as MMS is not without shortcomings it should not be applied indiscriminately. MMS may also be seen as a labor intensive feat, as patients often require anywhere from 1 to 6 rounds of resection for histologic clearance.[13] Other considerations include potentially requiring coordination between two surgeons, which can result in delays in executing treatment plans. Furthermore, as MMS is generally performed under local anesthesia, it becomes a nonviable option for larger tumors that require general anesthesia for more extensive surgical resection.

### Staged Excision

Last, staged excision entails resection of CM or NMSC followed by permanent section histologic assessment. Using formalin-fixed tissue has the disadvantage of a 24 to 48 hour delay in histologic

result but yields better quality sections, which can be processed using the automated systems of a histopathology laboratory. However, patients may require several procedures to obtain clear margins. Complex reconstruction should be deferred until clearance of permanent section margins, thereby requiring another surgical intervention and potentially appropriate wound care in the interim.

The standard treatment of invasive melanoma is with WLE (with or without sentinel lymph node biopsy depending on T stage) with delayed reconstruction. Delaying reconstruction can be seen as an inconvenience. However, it allows for definitive clearance of malignancy and allows the reconstructive surgeon time to develop a reconstructive plan and counsel patients.

One potential modality for obtaining permanent section analysis with melanoma in situ (MIS) is incorporation of the square procedure. MIS poses a particular challenge due to the propensity for subclinical extension beyond visible pigmented borders, potentially resulting in incomplete excision when adhering to National Comprehensive Cancer Network (NCCN) guidelines predicated on clear specimen borders.[14] In addition, the difficulty of differentiating the atypical melanocytic hyperplasia from chronically damaged skin exacerbates this problem. The staged square procedure entails excising a peripheral 2-mm wide strip of tissue corresponding to 100% of the peripheral margin for permanent vertical section margin analysis.[14] The resulting peripheral defect can then be sutured to surrounding wound edges, mitigating challenges with wound fibrosis or granulation bed bleeding during subsequent formal reconstruction.[14] A square procedure case of MIS in which there is significant subclinical extension of disease is illustrated in **Fig. 3**A–C.

Regardless of the resection modality chosen, mitigating the likelihood of positive margins and local recurrence is imperative to permit a subsequent safe reconstruction. The ability of the surgeon to produce a cosmetically and functionally adequate reconstruction would therefore be compromised if the primary reconstructive option was abandoned or irradiated due to the risk of residual disease. **Fig. 4**A, B shows the clinical challenge of managing a patient that was formally reconstructed before obtaining negative margins, thereby voiding a reconstructive option and clouding the ability to discern positive margin sites. This patient was ultimately referred to the senior author's practice (CLS) for treatment after she developed recurrent BCCs along the bilateral edges of the forehead flap.

## SKIN CANCERS

The reconstructive surgeon should possess a solid background knowledge of common cutaneous malignancies as disease treatment and risk of recurrence impacts reconstructive surgery.

### Melanoma

CM is the third most commonly diagnosed skin cancer in the United States.[6] Compared with NMSC, melanoma resections have higher local recurrence risk, greater degree of subclinical spread, and greater likelihood of requiring tissue rearranging reconstructive surgery.[15] Moreover, compared with trunk and proximal extremity CMs, those in the H&N subsites are two to three-fold more likely to have microscopic extension beyond the clinically visible tumor and are fivefold more likely to have positive margins after conventional excision.[15]

Owing to the aforementioned limitations of frozen section analysis, most CM has been treated with WLE. Margin recommendations for WLE are listed in **Table 1**.[16]

The risk of positive margins are higher in patients with advanced age, diagnosis via shave biopsy, lentigo maligna, or demosplastic subtypes, increasing tumor thickness, and presence of ulceration.[15] However, although NCCN guidelines acknowledge

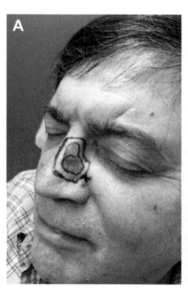
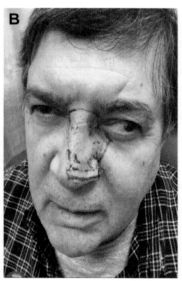
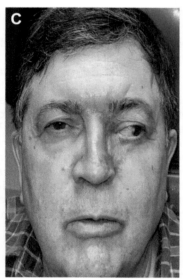

**Fig. 3.** (*A*) Patient with nasal melanoma in situ that had specimen and margin edges marked out using the square procedure. (*B*) After three-staged square procedures demonstrating the subclinical extension of melanoma in situ. (*C*) Followed by excision of diseased central island of tissue and skin graft reconstruction once negative margin status confirmed on permanent section analysis.

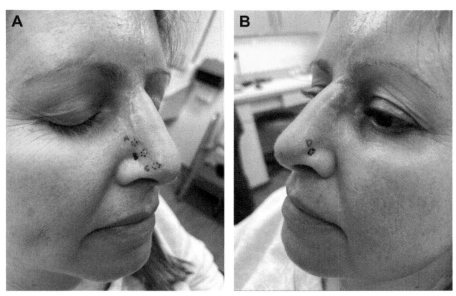

**Fig. 4.** (*A, B*) Patient with a nasal BCC that underwent excision and immediate forehead flap reconstruction at another institution with negative frozen section margins but positive permanent section margins later presented with recurrent malignancy along the edges of the flap.

peripheral resection margins may be modified to accommodate specific anatomic considerations, there is no prospective randomized assessment of this adaptation and narrower than recommended margins may increase the risk of persistent and recurrent disease. Furthermore, the NCCN maintains a strong preference to delay complex reconstruction until histologic margin assessment is complete due to the morbidity and difficulty of deconstructing complex reconstructions for further margin analysis. To date, there has not been a randomized trial directly comparing MMS with standard WLE or different forms of staged excision with permanent section analysis. MMS is not recommended as the primary treatment for invasive CM when standard clinical margins can be obtained.[12] The NCCN endorses permanent section analysis of CM as the current gold standard.

## Basal Cell Carcinoma

BCC is the most common type of skin cancer and the single leading cause of cancer among Caucasian individuals. The primary risk factors include increasing age, sun exposure, radiation exposure, fair skin, red or blond hair, light eye color, mutations of the *PTCH1* gene on chromosome 9q, and genetic syndromes including albinism, xeroderma pigmentosum, and nevoid BCC syndrome.

As BCC often possesses a highly favorable prognosis, minimizing morbidity becomes imperative with these skin cancers. Management for these relatively innocuous lesions can include cryosurgery, curettage, electrodesiccation, radiotherapy, and photodynamic therapy. However, these would not be considered primary interventions due to a lack of histologic confirmation of clearance. With respect to surgical margins, NCCN guidelines for low-risk BCC are 4-mm clinical margins. All BCC that occur on the nose are by definition high risk for local recurrence.[17]

An exception to standard WLE for BCC may be based on perioperative case-specific factors. Some higher risk features for poor prognosis within BCC include close or positive margins, tumor size $\geq$ 2 cm, poor tumor differentiation, perineural invasion (PNI), depth of invasion, and immunosuppression.[18] This has led to suggestions that with patients who possess high-risk features, there is a greater role of ensuring adequate resection via staged excision or MMS before reconstruction. Studies evaluating MMS versus WLE techniques for BCC have

| Table 1 | | |
| --- | --- | --- |
| **Recommended excision margins for melanoma based on tumor thickness** | | |
| **Tumor Thickness** | | **Recommended Margin** |
| Melanoma in situ | | 0.5–1.0 cm |
| $\leq$ 1.0 mm | | 1 cm |
| 1–2 mm | | 1–2 cm |
| $\geq$ 2 mm | | 2 cm |

demonstrated more favorable results with MMS, with local recurrence rates estimated at 3.1% and 14%, respectively.[19] In addition, systematic reviews have suggested lower recurrence rates in both primary and recurrent BCC cases following MMS.[20]

### Squamous Cell Carcinoma

Squamous cell carcinoma (SCC) is the second most common skin cancer, with more than 700,000 new cases diagnosed each year in the United States.[21] Prognosis remains excellent for the majority of cases, with a 95% cure rate with surgical excision.[22] Yet the discordance between frozen section and permanent margin analysis has been reported to be as high as 19.5%, with greater false-negative rates on frozen sections associated with poorly differentiated carcinoma, lymphovascular invasion, and PNI at 14%, 36% and 26%, respectively.[22]

As aforementioned, studies evaluating resection modalities within NMSC have demonstrated lower recurrence rates with MMS than those of WLE.[23] Specifically, studies have suggested cutaneous SCC managed with MMS yield a three times lower risk of recurrence relative to standard WLE after adjusting for tumor size and depth of invasion.[21] Moreover, MMS has been shown to yield smaller defects after resection in cutaneous SCC,[21] which in the nasal subunits may be the deciding variable between a local versus a more involved interpolated flap reconstruction.

Recent investigations of the NCCN stratification of cutaneous SCC into low, high, and very high-risk groups have reaffirmed the oncologic importance of surgical resection modality. Location on the nose is a high risk factor independent of tumor size. High and very high-risk cohorts demonstrate worse prognoses and therefore yield significantly improved outcomes of local recurrence, distant metastasis, and disease-specific death rates when MMS is the selected resection technique.[7] Similarly, nationwide prospective cohort studies have shown favorable incidence rates of recurrence at 1.3 and 4.5 per 100 person-years for BCC and SCC, respectively, following MMS.[24] Hence, the evidence to date favors MMS when managing high-risk cutaneous SCC.

## RADIATION

Previous exposure to radiation or future plans to radiate skin may impact reconstructive plans. Skin is particularly radiosensitive, with more than 95% of patients receiving radiotherapy developing moderate to severe skin reactions. In the acute phase, the skin typically becomes erythematous and may desquamate or ulcerate.[25] Acute damage usually resolves after therapy is completed, but chronic damage can develop months or years later and is collectively known as late radiation tissue injury. On the molecular scale, cytokine cascades and fibroinflammatory pathways are up-regulated due to radiation which can progress for many years leading to substantial fibrosis, the hallmark of chronic RT damage.[25] Late clinical manifestations include soft tissue fibrosis, skin atrophy, epithelial ulceration, skin necrosis, fistula formation, major vessel rupture, and impaired wound healing.[26] **Fig. 5**A, B shows late radiation changes to the nose including fibrosis, telangiectasias, nasal valve stenosis, and thinning of the epithelium.

For melanoma, adjuvant radiotherapy to the primary site of malignancy yields improved local control in high recurrence risk cases after surgery. Patients may have a combination of risk factors including H&N subsite, extensive neurotropism, pure desomoplastic histology, and close margins where re-resection is not feasible.[16] In the context of stage III melanoma, specifically as postoperative treatments after lymph node dissection, radiotherapy to the nodal basin may be indicated in select high-risk patients.[16]

For NMSC, similar high-risk features including deep invasion, lymphovascular invasion, size over 2 cm, poor differentiation, and PNI have been cited as indications for adjuvant radiotherapy.[27] In patients with extensive perineural or large nerve involvement, adjuvant radiotherapy may be effective in preventing local recurrence in the setting of surgery with negative margins.[28]

The contemporary literature evaluating the effect of adjuvant radiotherapy before or following nasal reconstruction on final functional and esthetic outcomes is scarce. From a practical point of view, the timing of immediate versus delayed reconstruction would be contingent on the possibility of clear oncologic resection, the characteristics of the final defect, and the complexity of the reconstruction. The American College of Surgeons and Commission on Cancer recently released the first quality metric for H&N oncology, wherein time to initiation of postoperative radiotherapy in surgically managed H&N SCC patients must be within 6 weeks.[29] As this is reflective of the robust evidence demonstrating worse oncologic outcomes with delayed initiation of postoperative radiotherapy, adherence to these recommendations is imperative. Thus, if a nasal defect requires a complex multilayered and multistaged reconstruction for definitive repair and it cannot be completed within the interval treatment window, a simple single-stage reconstruction can

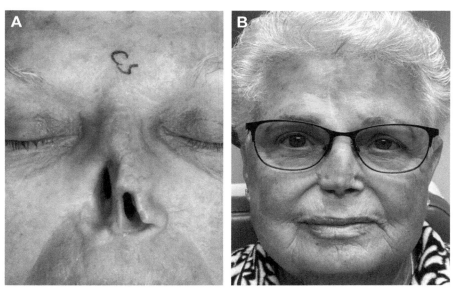

**Fig. 5.** (A) Patient with a nasal SCC who underwent partial rhinectomy and adjuvant radiation therapy. (B) Reconstructive outcome using a multistaged prelaminated forehead flap that was performed after the completion of adjuvant radiation.

be implemented with a formal reconstruction deferred until completion of adjuvant radiotherapy.

## PATIENT OUTCOMES

Patient self-reported questionnaires following facial skin cancer surgery have shown younger age, female sex, history of anxiety and/or depression, and nasal subsites as independently predictive of psychosocial distress.[5,30] Heightened anxiety about meeting new people is the persistent quality of life metric that does not seem to normalize by 3 months, illustrating the long-term social impact of facial reconstruction.[30] In evaluation of H&N melanomas, worse visual analog scale scores occurred with skin grafting compared with locoregional reconstruction.[31] In addition, patient-reported satisfaction scales have demonstrated decreased scores with lower nasal subunit defects and with primary closure as opposed to local flap reconstruction.[32] Hence, nasal tip defects warrant reconstruction by a surgeon with significant experience in this type of repair, even if it requires a brief treatment delay for referral.

## DELAYED RECONSTRUCTION

Historically, there was concern that delayed reconstruction may result in greater risk of infection as the wound is left open, requiring local wound care. However, literature to date has not suggested an increased risk of infection in

circumstances where reconstruction is delayed by a variable range from a few days to few weeks.[1,33] Studies estimate that delayed and immediate reconstructions yield comparable rates of minor infections which can vary on average from 4% to 9.3%.[1,33,34] Likewise, previous assumptions that delaying reconstruction in patients with comorbidities requiring anticoagulation or with diabetes mellitus causing greater rates of complication have not been demonstrated.[33] Similarly, there is no significant increased rate of perioperative bleeding or hematoma in patients with ongoing use of oral anticoagulants.[1] Delayed reconstruction may permit more time for patient counseling, shared decision-making for surgical plans, and preoperative consultations if these undertakings were not completed before resection.

From a physiologic perspective, delayed reconstruction has been demonstrated to improve full-thickness skin graft (FTSG) as well as composite graft viability, with those undergoing delayed reconstruction by a week or greater having lower likelihood of postoperative complications including graft failure.[35,36] Delaying graft placement allows the development of granulation tissue within the wound bed to enhance the optics of composite and skin graft survival beyond relying solely on plasma imbibition.[37,38] Other potential benefits of delayed grafting include better contour restoration from proliferation of granulation tissue, as well as smaller final defect size due to wound contraction and partial healing by secondary

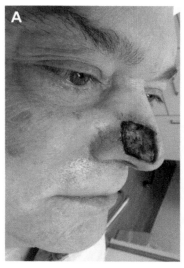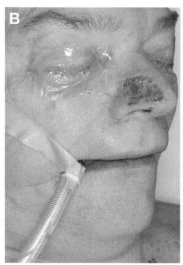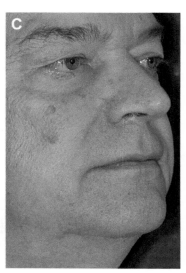

**Fig. 6.** (A) Nasal defect after excision of melanoma in situ, confirmed with permanent sections. (B) Two weeks of granulation. (C) After cartilage graft and full-thickness skin graft.

intention.[33] This physiologic postulation has been validated in previous studies comparing immediate versus delayed FTSG in nasal skin cancer following MMS, to demonstrate lower rates of partial graft loss in delayed grafting.[39] Likewise, delayed FTSG has demonstrated lower rates of nasal valve impairment and graft depression.[39] **Fig. 6**A–C demonstrates some of the aforementioned advantages of delaying reconstruction when cartilage or FTSG is planned.

Ultimately, if a more complicated repair or use of a composite graft is anticipated, or among active smokers, a delayed reconstruction for a period of 1 or 2 weeks may afford a greater likelihood of graft uptake due to the healthy granulation tissue bed.[35] Yet, reconstruction must still be performed with consideration of the overall timing to avoid sequelae once scar remodeling has begun. As wound contracture will plateau and scar will fill the remainder of the defect, the implications of specific nasal consequences such as alar notching must be considered.

One must be mindful of the fact that nasal defects tend to require the longest reconstruction time among the facial subunits, possess among the highest rates of complication, and more than 50% of incidences of facial reconstruction often require additional smaller modification procedures.[40] When comparing FTSG versus local flap reconstruction in NMSC, studies have demonstrated higher rates of hematoma and partial necrosis in patients undergoing skin graft reconstruction, with male sex and tumors above 15 mm size at a significantly higher risk of complication.[41] With respect to more intricate reconstructions, literature to date

corroborates full thickness or larger defects occupying multiple facial subunits, and those requiring composite grating or interpolated flaps carry a significantly higher risk of complication.[33,34] This is pertinent in nasal reconstruction as forehead flap reconstruction and auricular cartilage grafting is considered the workhorse of larger nasal tip defects.

## SUMMARY

Ultimately, literature to date does not clearly demonstrate the optimal time frame between resection and reconstruction. Inevitably, it falls on the clinician to consider the cutaneous malignancy at hand to select the appropriate timing of reconstruction. Subsequently, the patient-specific factors and reconstructive techniques used are cardinal variables in selecting the appropriate timing of repair.

## CLINICS CARE POINTS

- Complex reconstructive techniques after resection of cutaneous malignancy should ideally be used once negative margins are confirmed. If adjuvant radiotherapy is indicated, then reconstruction should not delay the initiation of radiation, which must start within 6 weeks of surgical resection.

- Delayed nasal reconstruction following skin cancer is not associated with higher risk of complication and may be a favorable decision when planning for full-thickness skin grafting, composite grafts, or interpolated flaps.

## DISCLOSURE

The authors have nothing to disclose.

## REFERENCES

1. Chen A, Albertini JG, Bordeaux JS, et al. Evidence-based clinical practice guideline: Reconstruction after skin cancer resection. J Am Acad Dermatol 2021;85(2):423–41.
2. Benkhaled S, Van Gestel D, Gomes da Silveira Cauduro C, et al. The state of the art of radiotherapy for non-melanoma skin cancer: a review of the literature. Front Med 2022;9:913269.
3. Bray HN, Simpson MC, Zahirsha ZS, et al. Head and neck melanoma incidence trends in the pediatric, adolescent, and young adult population of the United States and Canada, 1995-2014. JAMA Otolaryngol Head Neck Surg 2019;145(11):1064–72.
4. Liu S, Mathew P, Al Bayati M, et al. A cost analysis of Mohs and total surgical excision: a retrospective review of skin cancer treatments. Ann Plast Surg 2023; 91(1):e1–3.
5. Vaidya TS, Mori S, Dusza SW, et al. Appearance-related psychosocial distress following facial skin cancer surgery using the FACE-Q Skin Cancer. Arch Dermatol Res 2019;311(9):691–6.
6. Abrantes T, Robbins A, Kahn B, et al. Understanding melanoma in situ: Lentigo maligna surgical treatment terminology and guideline adherence, a targeted review. J Am Acad Dermatol 2023;S0190-9622(23):01084–8.
7. Stevens JS, Murad F, Smile TD, et al. Validation of the 2022 national comprehensive cancer network risk stratification for cutaneous squamous cell carcinoma. JAMA Dermatol 2023;159(7):728–35.
8. Moncrieff MD, Shah AK, Igali L, et al. False-negative rate of intraoperative frozen section margin analysis for complex head and neck nonmelanoma skin cancer excisions. Clin Exp Dermatol 2015; 40(8):834–8.
9. Mosterd K, Krekels GAM, Nieman FH, et al. Surgical excision versus Mohs' micrographic surgery for primary and recurrent basal-cell carcinoma of the face: a prospective randomised controlled trial with 5-years' follow-up. Lancet Oncol 2008;9(12):1149–56.
10. Muller FM, Dawe RS, Moseley H, et al. Randomized comparison of Mohs micrographic surgery and surgical excision for small nodular basal cell carcinoma: tissue-sparing outcome. Dermatol Surg 2009;35(9):1349–54.
11. van Kester MS, Goeman JJ, Genders RE. Tissue-sparing properties of Mohs micrographic surgery for infiltrative basal cell carcinoma. J Am Acad Dermatol 2019;80(6):1700–3.
12. Coit DG, Thompson JA, Albertini MR, et al. Cutaneous Melanoma, Version 2.2019, NCCN Clinical Practice Guidelines in Oncology. J Natl Compr Cancer Netw JNCCN 2019;17(4):367–402.
13. Van Coile L, Brochez L, Verhaeghe E, et al. A critical re-evaluation of Mohs micrographic surgery for a facial basal cell carcinoma in older adults: Should we waive this treatment in certain patients? J Eur Acad Dermatol Venereol JEADV 2023;37(9):1792–8.
14. Johnson TM, Headington JT, Baker SR, et al. Usefulness of the staged excision for lentigo maligna and lentigo maligna melanoma: the "square" procedure. J Am Acad Dermatol 1997;37(5 Pt 1):758–64.
15. Fix W, Etzkorn JR, Shin TM, et al. Melanomas of the head and neck have high-local recurrence risk features and require tissue-rearranging reconstruction more commonly than basal cell carcinoma and squamous cell carcinoma: A comparison of indications for microscopic margin control prior to reconstruction in 13,664 tumors. J Am Acad Dermatol 2021;85(2):409–18.
16. National Comprehensive Cancer Network. Melanoma: Cutaneous (Version 2.2023). Available at: https://www.nccn.org/professionals/physician_gls/pdf/cutaneous_melanoma.pdf. Accessed July 2023.
17. National Comprehensive Cancer Network. Basal Cell Skin Cancer (Version 1.2023). Available at: https://www.nccn.org/professionals/physician_gls/pdf/nmsc.pdf. Accessed July 2023.
18. Caparrotti F, Troussier I, Ali A, et al. Localized non-melanoma skin cancer: risk factors of post-surgical relapse and role of postoperative radiotherapy. Curr Treat Options Oncol 2020;21(12):97.
19. Dika E, Veronesi G, Patrizi A, et al. It's time for Mohs: Micrographic surgery for the treatment of high-risk basal cell carcinomas of the head and neck regions. Dermatol Ther 2020;33(4):e13474.
20. Alsaif A, Hayre A, Karam M, et al. Mohs micrographic surgery versus standard excision for basal cell carcinoma in the head and neck: systematic review and meta-analysis. Cureus 2021;13(11): e19981.
21. van Lee CB, Roorda BM, Wakkee M, et al. Recurrence rates of cutaneous squamous cell carcinoma of the head and neck after Mohs micrographic surgery vs. standard excision: a retrospective cohort study. Br J Dermatol 2019;181(2):338–43.
22. Chambers KJ, Kraft S, Emerick K. Evaluation of frozen section margins in high-risk cutaneous squamous cell carcinomas of the head and neck. Laryngoscope 2015;125(3):636–9.
23. Chren MM, Torres JS, Stuart SE, et al. Recurrence after treatment of nonmelanoma skin cancer: a prospective cohort study. Arch Dermatol 2011;147(5): 540–6.
24. Tomás-Velázquez A, Sanmartin-Jiménez O, Garcés JR, et al. Risk factors and rate of recurrence after mohs surgery in basal cell and squamous cell carcinomas: a nationwide prospective cohort (REGESMOHS, Spanish

registry of mohs surgery). Acta Derm Venereol 2021; 101(11):adv00602.

25. Borrelli MR, Shen AH, Lee GK, et al. Radiation-induced skin fibrosis: pathogenesis, current treatment options, and emerging therapeutics. Ann Plast Surg 2019;83(4S Suppl 1):S59–64.

26. Borab Z, Mirmanesh MD, Gantz M, et al. Systematic review of hyperbaric oxygen therapy for the treatment of radiation-induced skin necrosis. J Plast Reconstr Aesthetic Surg JPRAS 2017;70(4):529–38.

27. Yosefof E, Kurman N, Yaniv D. The role of radiation therapy in the treatment of non-melanoma skin cancer. Cancers 2023;15(9):2408.

28. Han A, Ratner D. What is the role of adjuvant radiotherapy in the treatment of cutaneous squamous cell carcinoma with perineural invasion? Cancer 2007; 109(6):1053–9.

29. Graboyes EM, Divi V, Moore BA. Head and Neck Oncology Is on the National Quality Sidelines No Longer—Put Me in, Coach. JAMA Otolaryngol Head Neck Surg 2022;148(8):715–6.

30. Zhang J, Miller CJ, O'Malley V, et al. Patient quality of life fluctuates before and after Mohs micrographic surgery: a longitudinal assessment of the patient experience. J Am Acad Dermatol 2018;78(6): 1060–7.

31. Buck D, Rawlani V, Wayne J, et al. Cosmetic outcomes following head and neck melanoma reconstruction: the patient's perspective. Can J Plast Surg J Can Chir Plast 2012;20(1):e10–5.

32. Veldhuizen IJ, Brouwer P, Aleisa A, et al. Nasal skin reconstruction: time to rethink the reconstructive ladder? J Plast Reconstr Aesthetic Surg JPRAS 2022; 75(3):1239–45.

33. Miller MQ, David AP, McLean JE, et al. Association of mohs reconstructive surgery timing with postoperative complications. JAMA Facial Plast Surg 2018; 20(2):122–7.

34. Patel SA, Liu JJ, Murakami CS, et al. Complication rates in delayed reconstruction of the head and neck after mohs micrographic surgery. JAMA Facial Plast Surg 2016;18(5):340–6.

35. David AP, Miller MQ, Park SS, et al. Comparison of outcomes of early vs delayed graft reconstruction of mohs micrographic surgery defects. JAMA Facial Plast Surg 2019;21(2):89–94.

36. Thibault MJ, Bennett RG. Success of delayed full-thickness skin grafts after Mohs micrographic surgery. J Am Acad Dermatol 1995;32(6):1004–9.

37. Lewis R, Lang PG. Delayed full-thickness skin grafts revisited. Dermatol Surg 2003;29(11):1113–7.

38. Moyer JS, Yang S. Optimal timing of reconstruction when using tissue grafts after mohs micrographic surgery. JAMA Facial Plast Surg 2019;21(2):94–5.

39. Robinson JK, Dillig G. The advantages of delayed nasal full-thickness skin grafting after Mohs micrographic surgery. Dermatol Surg 2002;28(9):845–51.

40. van Leeuwen AC, The A, Moolenburgh SE, et al. A retrospective review of reconstructive options and outcomes of 202 Cases Large Facial Mohs Micrographic Surgical Defects, Based on the Aesthetic Unit Involved. J Cutan Med Surg 2015;19(6):580–7.

41. Mamsen FPW, Kiilerich CH, Hesselfeldt-Nielsen J, et al. Risk stratification of local flaps and skin grafting in skin cancer-related facial reconstruction: a retrospective single-center study of 607 patients. J Pers Med 2022;12(12):2067.

# Approach to Major Nasal Reconstruction
## Benefits of Staged Surgery and Use of Technology

Heather K. Schopper, MD[a],*, Shekhar K. Gadkaree, MD[b],
Jessyka G. Lighthall, MD[a]

### KEYWORDS

- Nasal reconstruction • Hemirhinectomy • Subtotal rhinectomy • Complex facial defects
- 3D printing • Free flap reconstruction • Technology

### KEY POINTS

- In complex multi-subunit defects involving the nose and adjacent structures, the adjacent subunits should be reconstructed prior to nasal reconstruction.
- Anticipation of large nasal defects may allow for preparatory procedures like tissue expansion or prelaminated flaps.
- Technology like virtual surgical planning, 3 dimensional printing, and tissue engineering can help optimize outcomes for complex nasal defects.

## INTRODUCTION

While all defects on the face pose unique reconstructive challenges, large nasal defects are among the most challenging to approach. The nose is the central element of the face, providing an important aesthetic focus, while also serving an important functional role in the upper airway. Patients with significant nasal deformity face social stigmatization and challenges with breathing, exercise tolerance, olfaction, and support for glasses and masks.[1]

Given its prominence on the face, the nose is a very common site for sun-related skin cancers. While lesions may appear small initially, they can be more extensive than anticipated and result in large defects even when approached with Mohs micrographic surgery. Tumors can extend intranasally without clinical symptoms for some time or malignancies which originate sinonasally can extend superficially to involve the cartilage and skin.[2] In some practice settings, limited access to care or psychobehavioral comorbidities may lead to presentation at an advanced stage with large destructive masses that obliterate not only the structures of the nose proper but extend to involve the cheek, lip, periorbita, nasal bones, palate, or skull base.[3]

The structure of the nose is complex, made up of 9 distinct aesthetic subunits, 3 layers, and a framework composed of both bone and cartilage. The overall structural integrity of the nose relies upon the "L strut" composed of the caudal and dorsal septum and nasal cartilages including the upper and lower lateral cartilages. Portions of the nose, like the lateral ala, are solely supported by fibrofatty tissue but may require non-anatomic structural support in reconstruction. While the septal cartilage can be used as easily accessible graft material, in large defects, this cartilage may

[a] Division of Facial Plastic and Reconstructive Surgery, Department of Otolaryngology – Head and Neck Surgery, Penn State College of Medicine, 500 University Drive H-091, Hershey, PA 17033, USA; [b] Division of Facial Plastic and Reconstructive Surgery, Department of Otolaryngology – Head and Neck Surgery, University of Miami Miller School of Medicine, 1120 Northwest 14th St, Miami, FL 33136, USA
* Corresponding author.
E-mail address: hschopper@pennstatehealth.psu.edu

Facial Plast Surg Clin N Am 32 (2024) 199–210
https://doi.org/10.1016/j.fsc.2023.11.001
1064-7406/24/© 2023 Elsevier Inc. All rights reserved.

be insufficient or missing, requiring alternative autologous cartilage such as the ear or rib or the use of cadaveric donor tissue.[4]

The layers of the nose provide an additional reconstructive challenge. Unlike the cheek, there is little mobile skin on or adjacent to the nose which could easily be used as donor tissue for reconstruction of a large defect without risking significant distortion of adjacent structures. The framework of the nose must be reconstructed in 3 dimensions to provide support and contour, and the free structural grafts used in this framework require a bed of healthy vascularized tissue to survive. Perhaps the most troublesome layer of the nose to reconstruct is the lining of full-thickness defects. Intranasal mucosal flaps may be considered with smaller defects but subtotal or total rhinectomy defects leave little native tissue available for use and extensive framework that requires coverage.[5]

For all these reasons, the approach to major nasal reconstruction requires careful planning and consideration. Reconstruction can be particularly challenging in patients with multiple facial subunit involvement, scars from prior repairs, recurrent disease, aggressive or hard to clear disease, and those in need of adjuvant radiation. Repair is often approached in stages and technological resources like virtual surgical planning (VSP) and 3 dimensional (3D) printing are useful adjuncts when approaching these defects. There often is not a single correct answer when it comes to reconstruction and patient factors and goals play a large role in operative planning.

## DISCUSSION
### Multiple Facial Subunit Involvement

Large nasal defects often extend to involve the adjacent subunits including the cheek, upper lip, and orbit. In these cases, the sequence of reconstruction needs to be carefully considered in order to maximize function and survival of the reconstruction.

For all cases, reconstruction of surrounding subunits will be repaired prior to addressing the nasal defect to establish proper 3-dimensional (3D) position of the nose in relationship to the face. The medial cheek can often be repaired with local tissue advancement in older patients with greater skin laxity or by rotational advancement techniques like the cervicofacial flap in those with less redundancy. An upper lip defect can be approached in a similar fashion with primary closure for smaller defects as shown in **Fig. 1** or a variety of lip switch or complex rotational advancement flaps for larger defects. Co-existing cheek and lip defects may eliminate some nasal reconstructive options like a melolabial flap for alar reconstruction.[6] In cases of extensive loss of midfacial support, structural reconstruction with autologous bone flaps or implants is often required. When considering defects with associated orbital involvement, structural support for the medial orbit may need to be recapitulated prior to moving forward with nasal reconstruction to avoid migration of the globe and/or create a correctly sized and shaped orbit for prosthesis.

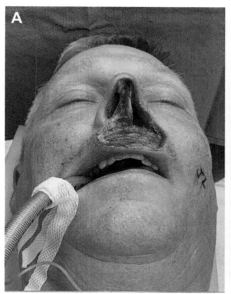 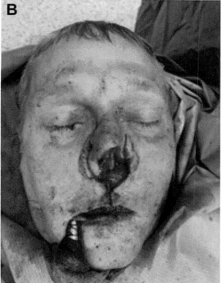

**Fig. 1.** (*A*) Combined lower third nasal and subtotal upper lip defect. (*B*) The lip was closed first to provide a base for the nasal reconstruction.

In many cases, these multi-subunit defects will require a staged approach, creating a base of healthy tissue around the nasal defect before proceeding with reconstructing the nose itself.

Another consideration with nasal defects may be associated resection of the anterior skull base. These resections, often performed in conjunction with neurosurgery, are challenging in and of themselves and often require at least partial reconstruction immediately if the dura is involved. An example is shown in **Fig. 2**. The approach to resection may include a coronal dissection which limits the ability to use workhorse flaps like the paramedian forehead flap. An inferiorly based pericranial flap is commonly used to repair large dural defects and is robust enough to withstand radiation. This does, however, eliminate the periosteum as a source of nasal lining in a laminated forehead flap.[7]

### Recurrent Disease or Prior Repair

Patients with recurrent disease or prior repairs are particularly challenging. Many of the most common reconstructive options may no longer be possible and a creative approach may be required. Advanced notice of resection can be helpful for planning with some preparatory measures taken prior to the ablative surgery if oncologically appropriate. In patients with prior paramedian forehead flap (PMFF), the contralateral side may be an option but the size of flap required and tissue laxity characteristics should be considered. In patients who will require a large amount of cutaneous coverage, tissue expansion may be an option as shown in **Fig. 3**.[8]

Grafting material options may also be limited. In patients with prior repair, septal cartilage may almost certainly be absent, as may auricular cartilage. In these settings, costal cartilage (autologous or cadaveric) or split calvarial bone grafts may be an option. Reconstructing the lining of the nose may be a particular challenge given the limited amount of mobile tissue available in the area at baseline. Some options in this case include a pericranial flap, a laminated free flap (**Fig. 4**), or a free flap with PMFF for skin reconstruction.[9–12]

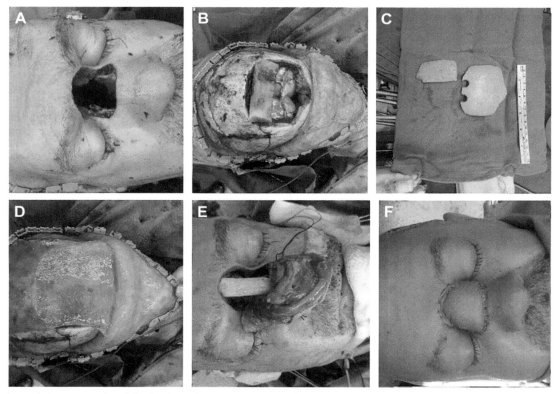

**Fig. 2.** (*A*) Upper and middle third nasal defect involving resection of the nasal bones and anterior skull base. (*B*) Anterior skull base defect exposed with dural onlay graft repair and bone flap removed. (*C*) Bone flap from frontal skull, part of which was used as bone graft for nasal dorsum reconstruction. (*D*) The pericranial flap was used to reconstruct the skull base and (*E*) a calvarial bone graft was used to reconstruct the nasal dorsum. (*F*) The structural reconstruction was wrapped in a radial forearm-free flap for both internal and external lining.

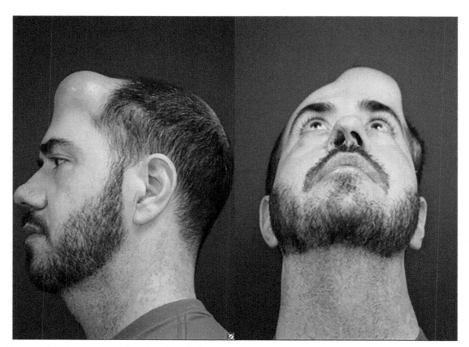

**Fig. 3.** Patient with prior paramedian forehead flap and recurrent disease of the right nasal ala. A 120 cc rectangular base tissue expander was placed in the forehead to recruit tissue for a repeat paramedian forehead flap prior to his planned resection. In this photo, patient still undergoing expansion prior to partial rhinectomy.

### Timing of Repair

Given the disfigurement associated with large nasal defects, the idea of immediate repair is attractive, but many factors should be considered regarding the timing of repair (**Table 1**). In some patients, the status of margins may not be clear at the time of resection or they may be at high risk for rapid recurrence due to aggressive disease. In these settings, it may be prudent to do a minimal repair immediately and delay more sophisticated work until the patient is known to be disease free lest early cancer regrowth destroy a complex repair effort. Medically fragile patients may not be suitable for the prolonged anesthetic time of a combined resection and repair.

The need for adjuvant radiation is a huge factor in timing of reconstruction. A classic concern with delayed repair, particularly in a field that will be radiated, is shrinkage of the soft tissue envelope and subsequent increased difficulty in repair. Radiated tissues have decreased elasticity, decreased perfusion, and increased risk of poor wound healing. Tissue planes are often distorted or obliterated, making dissection more difficult. Free grafts placed into radiated fields are at increased risk of necrosis and failure. On the other hand, radiation may cause a beautiful repair to fall apart over time and grafts to warp or become exposed. The reconstructive surgeon is then faced with the challenge of reconstruction in a radiated field with the additional handicap of a failed prior repair. Delayed repair also allows for completion of oncologic treatment with the tumor bed fully visible to assess for evidence of recurrence as shown in **Fig. 5**. Adjuvant treatment can be started without delay. A compromise between immediate and delayed repair may be a staged approach where vascularized tissue is transferred into the wound bed but section of the pedicle, graft placement, and refinements are performed after completion of and recovery from radiation.[13–15]

### Discretion in Extent of Repair

In an ideal world, every patient would be able to achieve near normal nasal structure and function after repair. As any reconstructive surgeon knows, this is far from the case. All of the earlier discussed factors go into the feasibility of repair, with the most important factor arguably being the patient's goals. In some settings, there is just not enough local tissue available for a more sophisticated repair or a patient may be too ill to undergo multiple stages and refinements. In these cases, a free flap for soft tissue coverage may be the appropriate choice even if it is not aesthetically ideal to provide wound closure and a significant amount of soft tissue that may be utilized for delayed repair.[16–19]

missed opportunity to utilize the armamentarium of the reconstructive surgeon, the aesthetic result can be impressive and patients can be extremely happy.[20] A prosthesis can also be an option for patients who have failed prior reconstructions or who are at high risk of recurrence with need to more easily surveil the sinonasal cavity. While the cost of prosthesis has been prohibitive for some patients, there are some prosthetic artists who are starting to accept commercial insurance. Advances in 3D printing may also hold some promise on this front.[21]

There are a number of options for type of prosthetics and means of retention as demonstrated in **Fig. 6**. The prosthetic can recapitulate part or all of the nose, with some designed for multi-subunit defects such as in orbital or palatal defects as well. They can be retained with adhesive, attached to glasses, or mounted to implanted posts similar to dental implants. When considering post placement, the risk of implant loss or hardware infection should be kept in mind, particularly in radiated beds.[22]

## Use of Technology

### Virtual surgical planning
VSP is an approach to reconstruction which utilizes computer-generated patient-specific models to provide the surgeon with an approach to the procedure which aims to optimize the aesthetic outcome while limiting the intra-operative time devoted to planning incisions or shaping hardware. This approach has been used for many years within the sphere of bony surgery; cutting guides for osteotomies are common in oncologic ablative surgery and osseous free flaps while virtual reduction of traumatic injuries is often used to develop pre-manufactured plates or plate bending guides. VSP services are often provided in conjunction with industry and utilize third-party engineers and proprietary software.

The use of VSP for non-rigid reconstruction is an emerging utilization of the technology. Soft tissue is easily deformable which makes modeling it much more challenging. The reliability of models may be affected by patient positioning, edema, pre-existing anatomic deformity, or imaging quality. This approach does, however, offer the opportunity to morph 3D models and create a perfected image as a goal for reconstruction or build constructs when multiple subunits are absent as shown in **Figs. 7** and **8**.[23,24] The perfected image can then be used to create a physical model for templating soft tissue flaps. This is a particular asset in complex 3D structures like the nose where estimating the tissue surface area required to

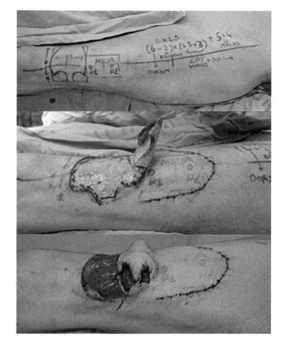

**Fig. 4.** Development of prelaminated anterolateral thigh-free flap for a combined total rhinectomy and medial cheek defect. The distal portion of the skin was used for the nose and the proximal for the cheek. The skin was raised in a suprafascial plane as the nasal skin layer. The fascia was then raised separately as the inner lining layer with a costal cartilage framework interposed between the 2 layers. From Bali and colleagues (2020),[11] used with permission.

Nasal protheses can also be an appealing option in patients who are either unwilling or unable to undergo the multiple surgeries required to refine a reconstruction. While this may seem like a

**Table 1**
**Pros and cons of repair before and after adjuvant radiation**

| | Pre-radiation | Post-radiation |
|---|---|---|
| Pro | • Limited duration of deformity for patient<br>• Sustain soft tissue envelope<br>• Well-vascularized bed | • Less risk if rapid disease recurrence<br>• No delay of adjuvant treatment if healing difficulties<br>• No potential for failed prior repair |
| Con | • Potential for hiding recurrence<br>• Possible repair failure/graft exposure after radiation | • Radiated tissue (less elasticity, less perfusion, obscured tissue planes)<br>• Risk of free graft failure<br>• Contracted soft tissue |

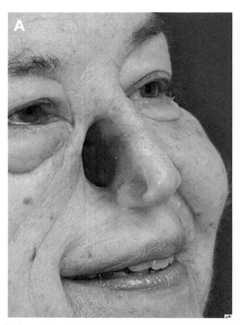 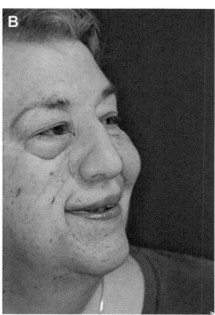

**Fig. 5.** Right hemirhinectomy defect in a patient with history of recurrent desmoplastic melanoma of the right nose with prior repair. After re-resection, she had a large combined cheek and nose defect. (*A*) The cheek defect was closed with local tissue advancement but the rhinectomy defect was left open for surveillance. (*B*) Adhesive-retained nasal prosthesis in place to cover the defect.

create alar contour or tip shape can be quite difficult and the contralateral side may be asymmetric or involved in the resection.[25]

The perfected images could also be used to develop nasal protheses that would rely less on the sculptural expertise of an artist, of which there are relatively few. As the technology progresses and modeling of the inherent deformational characteristics of the soft tissues and cartilage improves, this approach could be used to develop guides for framework cutting and incision planning.[26–28]

The reconstructive surgeon should keep in mind that VSP requires fine-cut patient imaging. This has likely been completed in the course of workup for extensive tumors or acute traumatic injuries but may not have been done prior to Mohs procedures or historical trauma. It may be advantageous to have pre-resection/injury images if the goal is creating a perfected soft tissue model. VSP is also relatively resource heavy and the relationships and infrastructure may not exist in all settings. Lead time for model building and delivery should be accounted for and forewarning of the need for repair would be helpful.

### 3D printing

3D printing is a technological adjunct to VSP and is growing in popularity, with many academic centers developing their own 3D printing labs in-house. Its use across medicine is broad, from developing custom prosthetic limbs, surgeon-specific instruments to bio-scaffolds for artificial organs. Within the realm of facial reconstructive surgery, 3D printed skulls are common in trauma and custom implants have been made for septal perforation reconstruction.[29] Stents for the nasal vestibule or internal nasal valve can be made to help with shaping of the reconstructed nose.[30–33]

This technology is rapid and customizable, with turn-around times as little as a day or 2 in settings with existing 3D printing set-ups. Relationships with bioengineers are required, as well as training with software and 3D printing machinery. In the time since this technology has come online, its accessibility has increased substantially with options for open source software and printers that are affordable enough for even home users. As with VSP, the source imaging needs to be considered when utilizing 3D printing. For patient-specific models, imaging is required and images acquired after resection or disfigurement will pose an additional modeling challenge. There are reports of the use of representative images from a database when patient-specific models were not possible.[34] Three D printing can also be used to make cutting guides for cartilage framework as shown in **Fig. 9.**[35] It should be kept in mind that 3D printed adjuncts are usually rigid or semirigid in nature

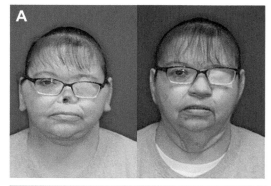

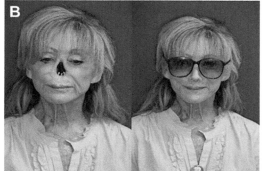

**Fig. 6.** Examples of nasal prostheses for subtotal and total nasal defects. (*A*) Patient with prior failed free-flap reconstruction requiring second free flap. Prosthesis is secured with adhesive. (*B*) Patient with multiple failed prior reconstructions. Magnetic prosthesis retained with implant. Adjunct procedures including lip lift and filler injections were used to help with prosthesis positioning and blend.

which can be helpful when they are used as structural models but may not be realistic when used to stand in for deformational tissues like the cartilages and soft tissues of the nose.

### Biocompatible materials

Major nasal reconstruction almost inevitably requires the use of graft material to recapitulate the structural framework of the nose. The most commonly used and easily accessible of these materials include septal cartilage, auricular cartilage, and costal cartilage. Other graft options include calvarial bone grafts, cadaveric rib, or osseous free tissue transfer. These options are often sufficient but very large subtotal or total rhinectomy defects may require the use of alternative biocompatible materials. While cutting guides could be made for autologous materials, the development of an extracorporeal framework can be complex and time consuming. In these settings, technology like VSP, 3D printing, and biocompatible polymers can be used to tandem to develop a framework.

When considering which material to utilize, the inherent nature of the nose should be considered. Rigid materials like metals would be unnatural and ceramics prone to fracture. Silicone is soft but may be too soft to provide support. The most commonly used biocompatible implants in this setting are biocompatible polymers. Porous polyethylene (Medpor®, Porex Surgical Inc, Newman, GA) has long been used in microtia repair, jaw augmentation, and midface implants. Manufactured dorsal implants, tip grafts, batten grafts, and nasal shells exist. Porous polyethylene allows for soft tissue ingrowth and graft incorporation which can be both an asset and a liability. Fracture of these grafts is a dreaded complication, as is infection and exposure. Other polymers like polycaprolactone and poly(L-lactic acid) have been used as implants and are easily printable.[36] Resorbable implants have also been used to maintain the soft tissue envelope and

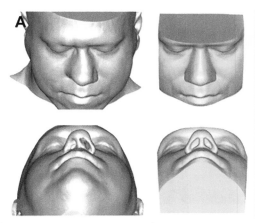

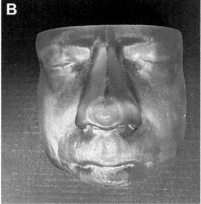

**Fig. 7.** (*A*) Pre-operative (gray) and perfected images (blue) generated in planning reconstruction for an anticipated hemirhinectomy defect in a patient with a prior paramedian forehead flap (PMFF). Generated in conjunction with Materialise and DePuy Synthes. (*B*) Printed model for use intraoperatively.

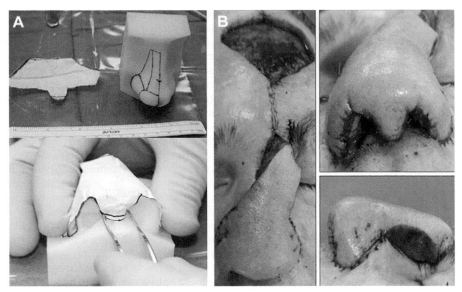

**Fig. 8.** (*A*) 3D printed model used to design template for PMFF. (*B*) The templated PMFF inset over the subtotal rhinectomy defect. (*From* Zeigler and Oyer (2021),[24] used with permission.)

nasal support in patients after near total septectomy with planned delayed reconstruction after radiation.[14,37]

Like all grafts, biocompatible implants require a healthy wound bed to decrease the risk of infection and implant extrusion so soft tissue flaps need to be planned. If no such wound bed is possible, repair should be considered in a staged fashion as outlined earlier prior to placing any non-native tissue in the field. If local soft tissue is insufficient to cover exposed bone, bio-scaffold material like Alloderm® (LifeCell Corp., Branchburg, NJ) or Integra® (Integra LifeSciences, Princeton, NJ) could be considered to encourage development of granulation tissue, mucosalization, or epithelialization in preparation for delayed reconstruction or prosthesis.

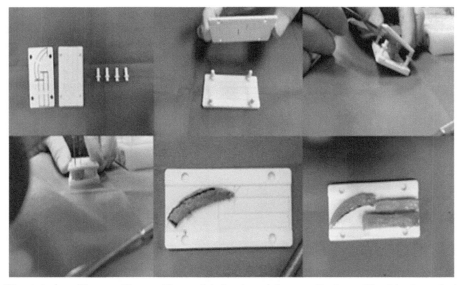

**Fig. 9.** A 3D printed cartilage cutting guide model developed from patient-specific virtual surgical planning. The guide was used to precisely carve costal cartilage when reconstructing a hemirhinectomy defect. (*From* Chiesa-Estomba et al (2022),[35] used with permission under Creative Commons international license CC BY 4.0.)

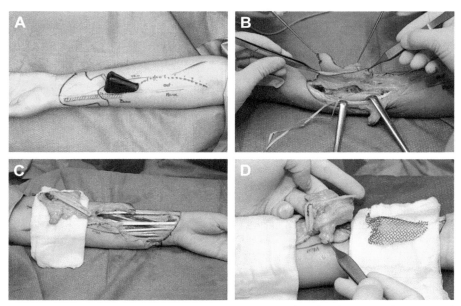

**Fig. 10.** Development of a laminated osteocutaneous radial forearm-free flap for a total rhinectomy defect. (*A*) A rubber model was used in planning. (*B-C*) The flap was raised with perforators intact. (*D*) The bone was then used to form the L strut framework and plated. The titanium mesh pictured was then laid between the bone and the skin to provide shape for the soft tissue. (*From* Ahcan and colleagues (2019),[42] used with permission under international license CC BY-NC 4.0.)

### Lab-grown autologous material

Perhaps the most sophisticated and patient-specific option for reconstruction of major nasal defects would be lab-grown autologous material. Tissue engineering is a booming field of medical research with work on-going regarding development of autologous nasal cartilage from patient stem cells and biocompatible frameworks. This could provide large volumes of graft material without the potential donor site morbidity for patients or the immunostimulatory potential of non-native tissue.[25,38] Most of the research on this front has been focused on repair of nasal septal perforations.[39,40]

This technology obviously requires a significant infrastructure and scientific expertise. Tissue engineering labs are often under the direction of a PhD investigator with extensive laboratory research expertise. The growth of patient cell populated graft requires donor cells which have to be harvested days to weeks before the intended reconstruction. This could be obtained at the time of biopsy of a suspect lesion or at the initial stage of a multiple stage reconstruction.[41]

The ultimate technological advance in nasal reconstruction would be the development of a complete nasal graft with a developed 3D structure and all 3 layers that would be inset with a microvascular anastomosis. The possibility of a complex lab-grown cartilage framework was initially developed in the infamous Vacanti mouse model, though to this day human trials of this technology have not come to fruition.[42]

### Patient Counseling

Perhaps the most critical component of reconstructive planning for major nasal defects is patient counseling. These situations are far from straightforward and pose a challenge to even the most experienced reconstructive surgeon. Patients very likely have little to no frame of reference for what such a complex reconstruction will look like or what their functional outcome could be. Elucidating their goals is critical; some patients' main goal may be to avoid multiple procedures and they may be willing to accept a suboptimal aesthetic or functional outcome. Others may want their nose to appear as close to normal as possible. In these conversations, they must be counseled about the likelihood for several surgeries over the course of months to years as well as the reality that even the best outcome will likely not be identical to their native nose. When considering a multistage approach, an intermediate stage for free cartilage graft placement or soft tissue thinning could be considered to optimize aesthetic outcome but prolongs a patient's time with an unsightly and sometimes distressing pedicle in the case of the paramedian forehead flap. Appropriate oncologic treatment should always be the primary goal. A patient's overall health needs to be taken into account, as does their ability to travel for multiple procedures and their network of friends and family for wound care and psychosocial support. Patients should be adequately prepared for their abnormal appearance and potentially compromised nasal airway in the interim repair stages which may affect their willingness or ability to perform their normal daily tasks. Finally, the idea of prosthetic rehabilitation to many seems like an inferior option to autologous tissue reconstruction. However, very nice aesthetic results may be obtained when a skilled anaplastologist is available.

### *Putting It All Together*

In cases of multi-subunit or total nasal defects, a multi-staged approach to autologous tissue reconstruction may provide optimal results. Careful patient counseling is critical in these cases as reconstruction may span many months with more than 3 stages. In these cases, a combination of VSP, model surgery, prelaminated free tissue transfer, and delayed structural reconstruction may be necessary such as in the case demonstrated by Ahcan and colleagues (**Fig. 10**).[43]

### SUMMARY

Reconstruction of large nasal defect with multi-facial subunit involvement, aggressive malignancies, need for radiation or wound bed monitoring, and cases of prior reconstruction are challenging for any reconstruction surgeon. A large number of factors may be considered when counseling patients, electing procedures to perform, and deciding when to perform them. Technological advances may assist in providing an optimal functional and aesthetic result and should be considered in complex cases.

### CLINICS CARE POINTS

- Thoughtful planning, including discussion with patients regarding their desires and willingness to undergo multiple procedures, is essential in the reconstruction of complex nasal defects.
- The pros and cons of reconstructing before or after radiation should be considered, particularly in patients with recurrent or aggressive disease.

- Smaller procedures before a larger reconstruction including tissue expansion and prelamination of flaps can optimize outcomes.
- Developing technology like 3D printing and VSP can be used creatively for planning and implementation of otherwise difficult to reconstruct defects.

### DISCLOSURE

The authors have nothing to disclose.

### REFERENCES

1. Andretto Amodeo C. The central role of the nose in the face and the psyche: review of the nose and the psyche. Aesthetic Plast Surg 2007;31(4):406–10.
2. Thawani R, Kim MS, Arastu A, et al. The contemporary management of cancers of the sinonasal tract in adults. CA Cancer J Clin 2023;73(1):72–112.
3. Panje WR, Ceilley RI. Nasal skin cancer:hazard to a uniquely exposed structure. Postgrad Med 1979;66(1):75–82.
4. Cannady SB, Cook TA, Wax MK. The total nasal defect and reconstruction. Facial Plast Surg Clin North Am 2009;17(2):189–201.
5. Joseph AW, Truesdale C, Baker SR. Reconstruction of the Nose. Facial Plast Surg Clin North Am 2019;27(1):43–54.
6. Jones NS, Raghavan U. Management of composite defects of the nose, cheek, eyelids and upper lip. J Laryngol Otol Suppl 2009;(32):1–38.
7. Racette S, Tekumalla S, Agarwal A, et al. Anterior Skull Base Reconstruction. Otolaryngol Clin North Am 2023;56(4):727–39.
8. Kroll SS. Forehead flap nasal reconstruction with tissue expansion and delayed pedicle separation. The Laryngoscope 1989;99(4):448–52.
9. Seth R, Revenaugh PC, Scharpf J, et al. Free anterolateral thigh fascia lata flap for complex nasal lining defects. JAMA Facial Plast Surg 2013;15(1):21–8.
10. Yen CI, Kao HK, Chang CS, et al. Simultaneous free flap and forehead flap for nasal reconstruction. Microsurgery 2023;43(5):470–5.
11. Bali ZU, Karatan B, Parspanci A, et al. Total nasal reconstruction with pre-laminated, super-thin anterolateral thigh flap: A case report. Microsurgery 2021;41(6):569–73.
12. Brunetti B, Tenna S, Barone M, et al. Bipaddle chimaeric forehead flap: A new technique for simultaneous lining and cutaneous reconstruction in case of full thickness defects of the nose. Microsurgery 2019;39(2):124–30.

13. Teichgraeber JF, Goepfert H. Rhinectomy: timing and reconstruction. Otolaryngology–head and neck surgery 1990;102(4):362–9.
14. Della Santina CC, Byrne PJ. Initial management of total nasal septectomy defects using resorbable plating. Arch Facial Plast Surg 2006;8(2):128–38.
15. McGuirt WF, Thompson JN. Surgical approaches to malignant tumors of the nasal septum. Laryngoscope 1984;94(8):1045–9.
16. Burget GC, Walton RL. Optimal use of microvascular free flaps, cartilage grafts, and a paramedian forehead flap for aesthetic reconstruction of the nose and adjacent facial units. Plast Reconstr Surg 2007;120(5):1171–207.
17. Salibian AH, Menick FJ, Talley J. Microvascular Reconstruction of the Nose with the Radial Forearm Flap: A 17-Year Experience in 47 Patients. Plast Reconstr Surg 2019;144(1):199–210.
18. Pinto V, Antoniazzi E, Contedini F, et al. Microsurgical Reconstruction of the Nose: The Aesthetic Approach to Total Defects. J Reconstr Microsurg 2021;37(3):272–81.
19. Gasteratos K, Spyropoulou GA, Chaiyasate K. Microvascular Reconstruction of Complex Nasal Defects: Case Reports and Review of the Literature. Plast Reconstr Surg Glob Open 2020;8(7):e3003. https://doi.org/10.1097/GOX.0000000000003003.
20. Becker C, Becker AM, Pfeiffer J. Health-related quality of life in patients with nasal prosthesis. J Craniomaxillofac Surg 2016;44(1):75–9. https://doi.org/10.1016/j.jcms.2015.10.028.
21. Denour E, Woo AS, Crozier J, et al. The Use of Three-Dimensional Photography and Printing in the Fabrication of a Nasal Prosthesis. J Craniofac Surg 2020;31(5):e488–91. https://doi.org/10.1097/SCS.0000000000006561.
22. Ethunandan M, Downie I, Flood T. Implant-retained nasal prosthesis for reconstruction of large rhinectomy defects: the Salisbury experience. Int J Oral Maxillofac Surg 2010;39(4):343–9. https://doi.org/10.1016/j.ijom.2010.01.003.
23. Zarrabi S, Welch M, Neary J, et al. A Novel Approach for Total Nasal Reconstruction. J Oral Maxillofac Surg 2019;77(5):1073 e1–e1073 e11. https://doi.org/10.1016/j.joms.2018.11.007.
24. Ziegler JP, Oyer SL. Prelmainated paramedian forehead flap for subtotal nasal reconstruction using three-dimensional printing. BMJ Case Rep 2021;14:e238146. https://doi.org/10.1136/bcr-2020-238146.
25. VanKoevering KK, Zopf DA, Hollister SJ. Tissue Engineering and 3-Dimensional Modeling for Facial Reconstruction. Facial Plast Surg Clin North Am 2019;27(1):151–61. https://doi.org/10.1016/j.fsc.2018.08.012.
26. Huang C, Zeng W, Chen J, et al. The Combined Application of Augmented Reality and Guide Template Technology in the Treatment of Nasal Deformities. J Craniofac Surg 2021;32(7):2431–4. https://doi.org/10.1097/SCS.0000000000007522.
27. Shi B, Huang H. Computational technology for nasal cartilage-related clinical research and application. Int J Oral Sci 2020;12(1):21. https://doi.org/10.1038/s41368-020-00089-y.
28. Sultan B, Byrne PJ. Custom-made, 3D, intraoperative surgical guides for nasal reconstruction. Facial Plast Surg Clin North Am 2011;19(4):647–53. viii-ix.
29. Rajzer I, Strek P, Wiatr M, et al. Biomaterials in the Reconstruction of Nasal Septum Perforation. Ann Otol Rhinol Laryngol 2021;130(7):731–7.
30. Cao Y, Sang S, An Y, et al. Progress of 3D Printing Techniques for Nasal Cartilage Regeneration. Aesthetic Plast Surg 2022;46(2):947–64.
31. De Greve G, Malka R, Barnett E, et al. Three-Dimensional Technology in Rhinoplasty. Facial Plast Surg 2022;38(5):483–7.
32. Jung JW, Ha DH, Kim BY, et al. Nasal Reconstruction Using a Customized Three-Dimensional-Printed Stent for Congenital Arhinia: Three-Year Follow-up. The Laryngoscope 2019;129(3):582–5.
33. Visscher DO, van Eijnatten M, Liberton N, et al. MRI and Additive Manufacturing of Nasal Alar Constructs for Patient-specific Reconstruction. Sci Rep 2017;7(1):10021.
34. Wei H, Zhang A, Tao C, et al. Three-Dimensional Rapid Printing-Assisted Individualized Total Nasal Reconstruction Based on a Database of Normal External Noses. Plast Reconstr Surg 2022;150(4):888–98.
35. Chisea-Estomba CM, Gonzalez-Garcia J, Sistiaga-Suarez JA, et al. A novel computer-aided design/computer-aided manufacturing (CAD/CAM) 3D printing method for nasal framework reconstruction using microvascular free flaps. Cureus 2022;14(9):e28971.
36. Hsieh TY, Dhir K, Binder WJ, et al. Alloplastic Facial Implants. Facial Plast Surg 2021;37(6):741–50.
37. Park SH, Yun BG, Won JY, et al. New application of three-dimensional printing biomaterial in nasal reconstruction. Laryngoscope 2017;127(5):1036–43.
38. Oseni AO, Butler PE, Seifalian AM. Nasal reconstruction using tissue engineered constructs: an update. Ann Plast Surg 2013;71(2):238–44.
39. Bagher Z, Asgari N, Bozorgmehr P, et al. Will Tissue-Engineering Strategies Bring New Hope for the Reconstruction of Nasal Septal Cartilage? Curr Stem Cell Res Ther 2020;15(2):144–54.
40. Rotter N, Aigner J, Naumann A, et al. Cartilage reconstruction in head and neck surgery:

comparison of resorbable polymer scaffolds for tissue engineering of human septal cartilage. J Biomed Mater Res 1998;42(3):347–56.

41. Oseni A, Crowley C, Lowdell M, et al. Advancing nasal reconstructive surgery: the application of tissue engineering technology. J Tissue Eng Regen Med 2012;6(10):757–68.

42. Vacanti CA. The history of tissue engineering. J Cell Mol Med 2006;10(3):569–76.

43. Ahcan U, Didanovic V, Porcnik A. A unique method for total nasal defect reconstruction – prefabricated innervated osteocutaneous radial forearm free flap. Case Reports in Plastic Surgery and Hand Surgery 2019;6(1):11–9.

# Decision Making in Nasal Reconstruction
## When to Use the Forehead Flap?

Virginia E. Drake, MD[a], Jeffrey S. Moyer, MD[b],*

KEYWORDS

- Forehead flap • Nasal reconstruction • Decision-making • Skin cancer reconstruction • Bilobed flap
- Skin graft

KEY POINTS

- The forehead flap is a mainstay for reconstruction of major nasal defects.
- Patient selection and discussion of preoperative surgical expectations are key.
- Studies on the psychosocial effects of major nasal reconstruction support complex reconstructive techniques, as the initial distress experienced by patients seems to resolve with time after completion of reconstruction.

## INTRODUCTION

Nasal reconstruction is a complex undertaking, and the functional and esthetic role of the nose requires a three-dimensional understanding of nasal structure and anatomy. For larger defects including a through-and-through defect, a three-layered reconstruction is necessary to reconstruct the outer skin, structural integrity, and internal lining of the nose. Adding to the complexity of the reconstruction, there is the paucity of surrounding donor tissue in the nose unlike other areas like the cheek or neck, where secondary movement from tissue is readily available to reconstruct the defect via a local flap with minimal distortion. The reconstruction must also balance preserving a patent airway and avoiding tissue bulk that may draw the eye toward tip or alar asymmetries. A reconstruction that is esthetically pleasing but functionally poor is not a successful result. Nasal subunits must be respected when planning the reconstruction, and that if more than a half of a subunit is resected, removal of the remaining subunit should be considered in order for incisions to follow esthetic lines.[1]

The entirety of the reconstructive ladder is available for nasal reconstruction; however, there is subunit specificity that should be considered depending on the characteristic of the defect. Although granulation/secondary intention is an option, some form of closure is often best except in the smallest of defects. Small defects may be treated with straight line closure (especially near the root of the nose where skin is less adherent to the underlying structures) or a skin graft. Small local flaps such a transposition or V-Y advancement flaps may also be appropriate. Structural additions such as auricular cartilage or septal cartilage grafts may be necessary to prevent nasal obstruction from alar collapse when the defect involves the lower third of the nose. Composite grafts from the ear also play an important role in the alar region as well as in the area of the soft tissue facet and columella. Larger defects may be addressed with local flaps or transposition flaps such as a bilobed flap or dorsal nasal flap which allow for secondary movement. With large and deep defects, the paramedian forehead flap is a surgical mainstay.

[a] Division of Facial Plastic and Reconstructive Surgery, Department of Otolaryngology–Head and Neck Surgery, University of North Carolina, 170 Manning Drive, CB #7070, Chapel Hill, NC 27599, USA; [b] Division of Facial Plastic and Reconstructive Surgery, Department of Otolaryngology–Head and Neck Surgery, University of Michigan, 1500 East Medical Center Drive; TC1904, Ann Arbor, MI 48109, USA
* Corresponding author.
E-mail address: jmoyer@med.umich.edu

Facial Plast Surg Clin N Am 32 (2024) 211–219
https://doi.org/10.1016/j.fsc.2024.01.002
1064-7406/24/© 2024 Elsevier Inc. All rights reserved.

The paramedian interpolated forehead flap (PMFF) is a reliable, pedicled flap that transfers tissue from the forehead to the nose (**Fig. 1**). It is unique in that it provides excellent nasal skin color and texture match and can provide multilayered closure with the turn-in technique[2] or along with a septal hinge flap, vestibular advancement flap, composite graft, or skin graft. The PMFF is based on a unilateral supratrochlear artery in addition to perforators of the proximal supraorbital artery.[3] The location of the supratrochlear artery is consistent, arising from the superomedial orbit medial to the supraorbital artery as a terminal branch of the ophthalmic artery, perforating the corrugator muscle, and entering the frontalis muscle 2 cm above the superior orbital rim. It then courses superiorly and becomes more superficial throughout the subcutaneous fat and skin of the forehead.[1] Surgically, the supratrochlear artery is located 1.7 to 2.2 cm off of midline and the flap is dissected in the subcutaneous or subgaleal plane until near the superior orbital rim where care is taken near the origin of the supratrochlear arteries.[4] Thinning or removing frontalis muscle in addition to back-cuts near the pedicle origin can increase the flap's reach. This is typically a two[5]- to three[6]-staged surgery, with the first stage involving the raising, thinning, and inset of the flap, with a possible intermediate step for continued contouring with the benefit of continued vascularized tissue. The final step is division of the pedicle 3 weeks after

inset,[7] and studies have sought whether even earlier separation is the most cost-effective and viable.[8,9] The pedicle is ligated, and the anatomic position of the eyebrow is restored.[10]

Although a PMFF is a standard and necessary procedure to reconstruct large nasal defects,[11] patients often have reservations about this surgery. In addition to concerns about a forehead scar, limitations on work and activities of daily living while the pedicle is in place can prove challenging for patient acceptance of the PMFF given the appearance of the flap during the initial stages of the procedure.[8] The attached pedicle is visually unappealing, does not allow for glasses to be worn,[12] and exposed tissue requires wound care which may necessitate help of another person, particularly in elderly patients or patients with physical or mental challenges.[13] These downsides and considerations are important to discuss and acknowledge. Identifying the patient's surgical goals is vital. To some patients, the esthetic result is worth these disadvantages, and here, the decision is easy to move forward with a PMFF. However, in other patients, with an appropriate defect, other less complicated, one-stage options may be reasonable alternatives to a PMFF.

In this review, the authors discuss when these clinical situations may occur and the considerations and requirements necessary for a successful reconstruction. Although some argue that a

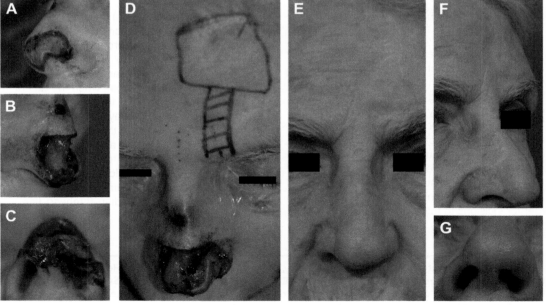

**Fig. 1.** Paramedian forehead flap defect and design. (*A*) Left oblique view of tip/alar defect. (*B*) Right-sided view of tip/supratip defect. (*C*) Base view of the defect. Note the addition of auricular cartilage onto the left lower lateral cartilage for structural support. (*D*) Design of the PMFF. (*E*) Frontal view of healed result and forehead scar. (*F*) Right oblique view of healed PMFF. (*G*) Base view of PMFF.

forehead flap should not necessarily be a patient "choice,"[1] the authors suggest that by keeping in mind a patient's priorities in conjunction with careful evaluation of the defect, there are often times where shared decision making may allow for alternative reconstructive options in lieu of a PMFF.

## DISCUSSION
### Patient Selection: "Decision Points"

On initial patient evaluation for nasal reconstruction, the first and most critical goal is to define the patient's surgical goals. To some patients who are more esthetically minded, they may be willing to undergo whatever is necessary for the most natural appearing result. Others may express that their priorities are for a straightforward reconstruction, with less emphasis on the cosmetic consequences. These priorities exist on a spectrum, so a candid discussion of the benefits and disadvantages of reconstructive options is essential. Other elements to consider include an evaluation of medical comorbidities including pulmonary or cardiac ability to tolerate general anesthesia or sedation, use of anticoagulant or antiplatelet medications, or wound healing impairing factors including poorly controlled diabetes or current smoking. The presence of quickly recurrent nasal malignancies or other aggressive lesions of the nose may also affect the reconstructive method used and may sway a surgeon toward a more conservative approach until they are addressed. However, given the straightforward harvest and limited anatomic dissection of the PMFF, even patients on anticoagulation/antiplatelet agents or with severe comorbid disease or advanced age can tolerate the surgery without hemodynamic issues intraoperatively.[1] In particular, a PMFF can be performed under local anesthesia in a treatment room if the patient is accepting of this approach and capable of sitting still for an extended period of time until the procedure is completed. The defect itself should be carefully examined: defect depth, evidence of intact perichondrium, proximity to the alar rim, and subunits involved are all important factors. The height of patient's forehead hairline also helps guide whether a patient might expect hair-bearing skin on the reconstruction if a PMFF were to be used.

### Indications for a Paramedian Forehead Flap

In most cases, the indication for a PMFF is straightforward: a large, deep, or full-thickness defect or in the setting of near-total or total nasal reconstruction.[11] Larger defects that involve the alar margin are also frequently best suited for a PMFF given the risk of alar retraction or collapse.

In these situations, a forehead flap is the most ideal option to restore nasal form and function. Here, the decision-making process is fairly straightforward. In hesitant patients, excellent communication, preoperative education with preoperative and postoperative photographs, assurance of perioperative support of friends or family, and careful perioperative and postoperative care are essential in helping them through the reconstructive process. Appropriate counseling and education is essential to assist patients through their multistage reconstruction.

### Forehead Flap Versus Skin Graft

Although the consideration of skin graft in the same setting of a forehead flap may seem contradictory, in select patients with specific goals and with a particular superficial nasal defect, a skin graft may represent a viable option for those who desire to avoid a forehead flap.[14] For example, a patient who is willing to accept some color mismatch of the nose to avoid a forehead scar or who is not medically able to tolerate a longer surgery but is willing to accept some contour irregularity as long as function is not impaired, a full-thickness skin graft may provide an acceptable option.[15]

For a skin graft to be considered, the defect needs to have an amenable recipient bed and have the appropriate underlying soft tissue structural support. For example, in a more superficial yet larger diameter defect, like that seen in resection of lentigo maligna melanoma in situ, this may be the case. Perichondrium would ideally be intact and the defect depth should be fairly minimal. Sometimes, allowing natural granulation over a few weeks demonstrates that even a deeper defect can reduce its depth via secondary healing and may be appropriate for a skin graft.[16]

However, caution should be taken in how a skin graft may contract and potentially distort the nasal ala. In these situations, an auricular cartilage graft along with the full-thickness skin graft can help both with alar support as well as volume of the defect[17] (**Fig. 2**). Color mismatch may also be an issue,[18] as it may appear "patch-like" especially in the setting of sebaceous, erythematous, or rosacea-prone skin (**Fig. 3**). In these scenarios, discussion of expectations with the patient is critical. In the right defect, a full-thickness skin graft does not "burn bridges," and if a patient is not satisfied with the outcome, a paramedian forehead flap can be performed secondarily, though in our experience this is rarely, if ever, needed.

Assessment of an individual's desire for an optimal esthetic outcome in a patient willing and able to undergo multistage surgery should steer a

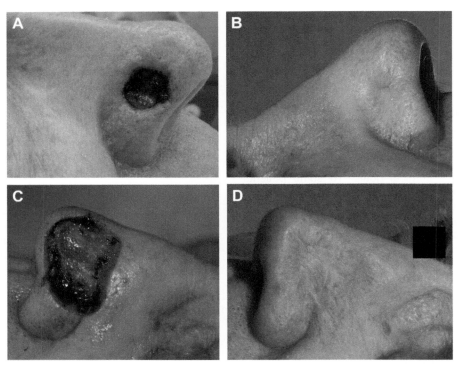

**Fig. 2.** Examples of full-thickness skin graft with auricular cartilage for larger nasal defects. (*A*) Right alar defect of Patient 1. (*B*) Patient 1 status post full-thickness skin graft (FTSG) with auricular cartilage graft (ACG). (*C*) Patient 2 with a larger left alar/tip/supratip defect. (*D*) Patient 2 status post-FTSG with ACG.

surgeon toward a PMFF. However, in the ideal defect and with a patient's priorities aligned with a single-staged reconstruction, a full-thickness skin graft on a larger, more superficial or secondarily-healed defect will save the patient the morbidity of a forehead flap.

### Forehead Flap Versus Local Flap (i.e., Bilobed Flap)

Another decision point is whether to use a local flap, such as a bilobed flap, instead of a PMFF.

In select cases, when a defect is deeper and a full-thickness skin graft would likely create a significant contour deformity and is generally 1.5 cm or less, a bilobed flap can be considered (**Fig. 4**).[19] The bilobed flap can be based medially or laterally and takes advantage of the secondary tissue movement from the nasal sidewall where skin is thinner, more lax, and less adherent in order to provide for coverage of supratip and tip defects.[20] The ideal defect is in the tip or supratip region, though medial alar defects, sidewall, and dorsal defects may also be appropriate for a bilobed

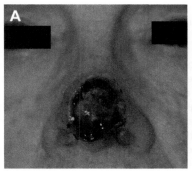 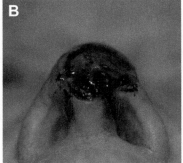 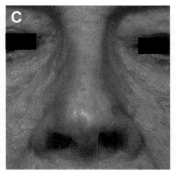

**Fig. 3.** Demonstration of hypopigmented FTSG. Columellar, soft tissue triangle, and tip defect. (*A*) Frontal view of defect. (*B*) Basal view of defect. (*C*) Status post full-thickness skin graft. Example of the challenge of color mismatch with the FTSG.

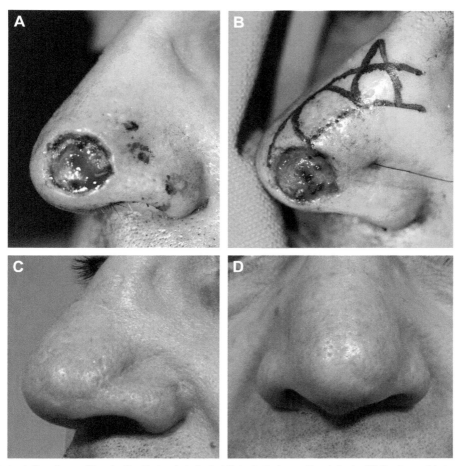

**Fig. 4.** Bilobed flap for a "Borderline" sized defect. (*A*) Left tip/supratip defect. (*B*) Design of laterally based bilobed flap. (*C*) Left oblique view of healed bilobed flap. (*D*) Frontal view of healed bilobed flap.

flap. The defect needs to be far enough from the alar rim or soft tissue facet to prevent alar retraction.[21] The patient's nose must be anatomically large enough to provide the appropriate soft tissue movement and skin availability, as a small nose may not be able to provide enough tissue for a 1.5 cm defect.[22] With wide undermining of the entire nasal superficial musculoaponeurotic system and precise flap design, the surgeon can often reconstruct "borderline" defects with a bilobed flap in defects where traditionally a PMFF would be used. The bilobed may risk raising the tip or ala and distorting other areas of the nose if undermining is not sufficient and/or the defect is excessively large. Additional nasal scars are introduced due to the flap design; however, incisions are limited to the nose. Using adjacent tissue avoids the color mismatch of a skin graft.

A study comparing the bilobed and the forehead flap with both scar assessment scores and three-dimensional optical scans found that reconstructive outcomes were not significantly different between the reconstructive modalities. Not surprisingly, the greatest clinical difference found between the two flaps was that the paramedian forehead flap was used for larger defects.[23]

## Psychosocial Considerations

Although to the surgeon a forehead flap is a routine procedure that yields consistent and excellent reconstructive results, patients are often wary of this reconstructive approach. The multistaged nature and time with the attached pedicle means that they may be unable to participate in work or daily activities. This consideration is significant and is meaningful to patients who may feel disfigured for several weeks awaiting the next surgical stage.[24] Although it is important to take the patient's goals and expectations for surgery into account, psychosocial considerations are also important in determining the best reconstructive approach.

Pepper and colleagues[25] surveyed 59 patients undergoing nasal reconstruction (including 14 interpolated flaps) via the Derriford Appearance Scale,[24,26] a 24-item survey which delineates patients' distress related to their appearance. Regardless of reconstruction method (skin graft, local flap, or interpolated flap), levels of distress were significantly higher at their postoperative visit for all patients. During this first visit, those who underwent an interpolated flap did have significantly higher levels of distress compared with cohorts who underwent full-thickness skin graft. However, at later follow-up (>12 weeks), the distress differential between those who underwent interpolated flap and skin graft was no longer different and became equivalent among the groups. This demonstrates that the mode and complexity of reconstruction does not have long-lasting psychosocial effects. Those who do undergo PMFF are expected to have increased levels of distress given the visibility and care required of their surgical sites while awaiting detachment, but in time this lessens. Timing also likely plays a part in quality of life after nasal reconstruction, as completion of the reconstruction within 6 months is associated with better quality of life.[27]

Another group[28] used the Derriford Appearance Scale in addition to a few other measures including the Brief Fear of Negative Evaluation Score[29] for 48 patients who underwent PMFF. The patients were stratified by defect severity into the number of nasal subunits involved in the reconstruction. As expected, social avoidance and distress measures were high immediately after surgery which then decreased after flap division or adjuvant procedures. The time point in the reconstructive process was associated with the level of psychosocial distress. This study supports the concept that despite the immediate anxiety, the PMFF may cause in time; this improves in sync with the healing process.

Surveys can also help identify those who are at greater risk of psychosocial distress during major nasal reconstruction. Vaidya and colleagues[30] used the FACE-Q Skin cancer survey and found that younger patients, those who had surgery on their nose, and a history of depression or anxiety scored higher in the self-consciousness and unhappiness domains in the first 3 months following surgery and were independent risk factors with distress. The psychological distress scores improved over time, however, self-consciousness persisted through the postoperative period.[30] Despite the psychosocial distress associated with a major nasal reconstruction process, the PMFF technique has been associated with high satisfaction in quality of life measures and functional outcomes.[27]

It is the nature of the PMFF to increase patient-related distress during the time of reconstruction, which eventually dissipates as the final result is realized and healing is completed. However, the best way to optimize patient satisfaction is by setting patient preoperative expectations, ensuring good communication, and initiating in-depth preoperative discussion for a team-driven approach to the reconstruction.

## Preoperative Preparation and Postoperative Expectations

Studies have been performed on the importance and value of standardized wound care protocols and resources for Mohs micrographic surgery (MMS), although the importance of this in the setting of a forehead flap has not been robustly evaluated. One study showed that preoperative educational materials improved patient comprehension before forehead flap surgery.[31] In-person education remains a gold standard of preoperative communication that best addresses patient's needs and questions[32] (ie, "What should I buy before the procedure? How do I take care of the pedicle?"). Of note, most research on how best to institute patient education has been performed during a patient's initial MMS, but there is a paucity of best practices in how to better the patient's reconstructive experience, and represents an area for further study in the facial plastic and reconstructive field.

A preoperative phone call 1 week before MMS did not improve satisfaction in patients,[33] though postoperative telephone calls do improve patient anxiety.[34] Other methods for patient communication and education include online modules[35] or communication like postoperative text messaging,[36] which lessened patient anxiety by 19%. Although multiple modalities allow for flexibility and increased access for postoperative questions, the in-person consultation and visit with the surgeon or a nurse educator are critical.[32]

In the authors' experience, the preoperative visit with the surgeon can be combined with time spent with a nurse educator who can discuss wound care and expectations in detail with written instructions that are available online as well. The use of photographs that clearly demonstrate what the patient will experience during the perioperative period are essential so that they can mentally prepare for the 3 or more weeks that the flap is in place. Having patients understand the final result is also important for the acceptance of the PMFF. In addition, showing patients what are common results with skin grafts and color mismatch as well as incisions for the bilobed flap are also helpful for tailoring discussions of what is most appropriate for any given patient. Discussing expectations is essential, and discussing common postoperative concerns like pain control, how to wear glasses, and the expected oozing, crusting, care of the pedicle and incisions, and other topics unique to the PMFF should be addressed. Addressing whether primary closure of the forehead defect is expected depending on the size of the nasal defect also allows for a comprehensive evaluation of "what to expect" which is best discussed preoperatively rather than postoperatively. With a thorough preoperative discussion, issues that arise are not an afterthought, but are expected avenues that may be encountered; the patient's mental preparation is key to good patient–surgeon communication and postoperative satisfaction.

Another aspect of the reconstructive process that can be discussed with patients preoperatively is the potential need for laser, dermabrasion, laser hair removal,[37] or scar revision.[38] Especially in patients with rosacea or sebaceous skin,[39] a fractionated or ablative laser[40,41] helps to obtain color and texture match of the forehead flap. Preemptive discussion of these options with patients in order to better the cosmetic result demonstrates the surgeon's eye for esthetic goals and willingness to continue to follow them after the immediate postoperative period to ensure the best possible functional and esthetic result.

## Viewing the Defect

In our clinical experience, occasionally patients ask not to view their post-Mohs defect before reconstruction. However, Veldhuizen and colleagues[42] argue that patient viewing of the defect is an important part of the reconstructive process. The patient should see where they have started to understand their progress. This helps set expectations appropriately which is key in managing patient satisfaction. This study evaluated whether there was difference in patient satisfaction if they looked in the mirror before reconstruction. A patient's view and appraisal of their scar changed when they looked in the mirror preoperatively. Specifically, female patients who looked in the mirror beforehand had higher satisfaction with their scar and reconstructive outcome. Those who viewed their defect before their reconstruction experienced overall less distress related to their reconstruction. The authors urge surgeons to encourage patients to view their defect preoperatively as a communication tool, as the complexity or the need for a forehead flap should be seen as necessary step to ensure mutual understanding between patient and surgeon.[42]

## SUMMARY

The PMFF is an essential modality in the reconstructive ladder for nasal reconstruction. In select situations—with the right patient and the right defect—a skin graft (with or without cartilage) or a bilobed flap can be considered for defects that some reconstructive surgeons might consider most appropriate for a PMFF. Although patients experience some level of distress with major nasal reconstruction, this subsides in time as the reconstruction matures. Encouraging a patient to view their defect is an important communication tool which can help patients better understand reconstructive needs. Excellent preoperative education with preoperative and postoperative photographic results, expectation-setting, and postoperative communication if questions arise is key to ensuring patient satisfaction.

## CLINICS CARE POINTS

- Nasal reconstruction requires careful evaluation of the defect alongside assessment of the patient's goals.
- Local flaps and full-thickness skin grafts can be considered for larger defects in select situations.
- Preoperative viewing of a cutaneous defect is beneficial as it helps patients understand the "starting point" of their reconstruction.
- Regardless of technique, nasal reconstruction is likely to cause most patients distress in the acute period, which then improves over time.

## DISCLOSURE

The authors have nothing to disclose.

## REFERENCES

1. Correa BJ, Weathers WM, Wolfswinkel EM, et al. The forehead flap: the gold standard of nasal soft tissue reconstruction. Semin Plast Surg 2013;27(2): 96–103.
2. Menick FJ. A new modified method for nasal lining: the Menick technique for folded lining. J Surg Oncol 2006;94(6):509–14.
3. Oleck NC, Hernandez JA, Cason RW, et al. Two or three? approaches to staging of the paramedian forehead flap for nasal reconstruction. Plast Reconstr Surg Glob Open 2021;9(5):e3591.
4. Shumrick KA, Smith TL. The anatomic basis for the design of forehead flaps in nasal reconstruction.

Arch Otolaryngol Head Neck Surg 1992;118(4): 373–9.

5. Menick FJ. Nasal reconstruction with a forehead flap. Clin Plast Surg 2009;36(3):443–59.

6. Menick FJ. A 10-year experience in nasal reconstruction with the three-stage forehead flap. Plast Reconstr Surg 2002;109(6):1839–55. discussion 1856-1861.

7. Shaye DA, Tollefson TT. What Is the optimal timing for dividing a forehead flap? Laryngoscope 2020; 130(10):2303–4.

8. Calloway HE, Moubayed SP, Most SP. Cost-effectiveness of Early Division of the Forehead Flap Pedicle. JAMA Facial Plast Surg 2017;19(5):418–20.

9. Rudy SF, Abdelwahab M, Kandathil CK, et al. Paramedian forehead flap pedicle division after 7 days using laser-assisted indocyanine green angiography. J Plast Reconstr Aesthetic Surg 2021;74(1): 116–22.

10. Yalamanchali S, Alvi SA, Hamill CS, et al. Eyebrow position after paramedian forehead flap nasal reconstruction. JAMA Facial Plast Surg 2019;21(1):79–81.

11. Menick FJ. Forehead flap: master techniques in otolaryngology-head and neck surgery. Facial Plast Surg 2014;30(2):131–44.

12. Qu LT, Kelpin JP, Eichhorn MG, et al. Spectacles under pedicles: eyewear modification with the paramedian forehead flap. Plast Reconstr Surg Glob Open 2016;4(8):e1003.

13. Chen CL, Most SP, Branham GH, et al. Postoperative complications of paramedian forehead flap reconstruction. JAMA Facial Plast Surg 2019;21(4): 298–304.

14. Weathers WM, Bhadkamkar M, Wolfswinkel EM, et al. Full-thickness skin grafting in nasal reconstruction. Semin Plast Surg 2013;27(2):90–5.

15. Gloster HM. The use of full-thickness skin grafts to repair nonperforating nasal defects. J Am Acad Dermatol 2000;42(6):1041–50.

16. Robinson JK, Dillig G. The advantages of delayed nasal full-thickness skin grafting after Mohs micrographic surgery. Dermatol Surg 2002;28(9):845–51.

17. Zopf DA, Iams W, Kim JC, et al. Full-thickness skin graft overlying a separately harvested auricular cartilage graft for nasal alar reconstruction. JAMA Facial Plast Surg 2013;15(2):131–4.

18. Segawa Y, Tono H, Chiba H, et al. Case series of modified dermis graft for skin defects of the nasal region. J Dermatol 2022;49(12):1330–3.

19. Okland TS, Lee YJ, Sanan A, et al. The bilobe flap for nasal reconstruction. Facial Plast Surg 2020; 36(3):276–80.

20. Steiger JD. Bilobed flaps in nasal reconstruction. Facial Plast Surg Clin North Am 2011;19(1):107–11.

21. Cook JL. Reconstructive utility of the bilobed flap: lessons from flap successes and failures. Dermatol Surg 2005;31(8 Pt 2):1024–33.

22. Losco L, Bolletta A, Pierazzi DM, et al. Reconstruction of the nose: management of nasal cutaneous defects according to aesthetic subunit and defect size. A Review. Medicina (Kaunas) 2020;56(12):639.

23. Peters F, Mücke M, Möhlhenrich SC, et al. Esthetic outcome after nasal reconstruction with paramedian forehead flap and bilobed flap. J Plast Reconstr Aesthetic Surg 2021;74(4):740–6.

24. Koster ME, Bergsma J. Problems and coping behaviour of facial cancer patients. Soc Sci Med 1990;30(5):569–78.

25. Pepper JP, Asaria J, Kim JC, et al. Patient assessment of psychosocial dysfunction following nasal reconstruction. Plast Reconstr Surg 2012;129(2): 430–7.

26. Carr T, Moss T, Harris D. The DAS24: a short form of the Derriford Appearance Scale DAS59 to measure individual responses to living with problems of appearance. Br J Health Psychol 2005;10(Pt 2):285–98.

27. Pagotto VPF, Tutihashi RMC, Ribeiro RDA, et al. Application of Face-Q and nose in nasal reconstruction with paramedian frontal flap after skin cancer resection. Plast Reconstr Surg Glob Open 2021; 9(4):e3533.

28. Yen CI, Su YJ, Chang CS, et al. Forehead flap reconstruction in different nasal defect: 58 patients' psychological outcomes. J Craniofac Surg 2023;34(5): 1387–92.

29. Collins KA, Westra HA, Dozois DJA, et al. The validity of the brief version of the Fear of Negative Evaluation Scale. J Anxiety Disord 2005;19(3):345–59.

30. Vaidya TS, Mori S, Khoshab N, et al. Patient-reported aesthetic satisfaction following facial skin cancer surgery using the FACE-Q skin cancer module. Plast Reconstr Surg Glob Open 2019;7(9):e2423.

31. Krane NA, Smith JB, Fassas S, et al. Educational materials improve patient comprehension in forehead flap surgery. Facial Plast Surg Aesthet Med 2021;23(6):489–90.

32. Patel P, Malik K, Khachemoune A. Patient education in Mohs surgery: a review and critical evaluation of techniques. Arch Dermatol Res 2021;313(4):217–24.

33. Sobanko JF, Da Silva D, Chiesa Fuxench ZC, et al. Preoperative telephone consultation does not decrease patient anxiety before Mohs micrographic surgery. J Am Acad Dermatol 2017;76(3):519–26.

34. Hafiji J, Salmon P, Hussain W. Patient satisfaction with post-operative telephone calls after Mohs micrographic surgery: a New Zealand and U.K. experience. Br J Dermatol 2012;167(3):570–4.

35. Migden M, Chavez-Frazier A, Nguyen T. The use of high definition video modules for delivery of informed consent and wound care education in the Mohs Surgery Unit. Semin Cutan Med Surg 2008; 27(1):89–93.

36. Hawkins SD, Koch SB, Williford PM, et al. Web app- and text message-based patient education in Mohs

micrographic surgery-a randomized controlled trial. Dermatol Surg 2018;44(7):924–32.

37. Ci Y, Cj C, Cs C, et al. Laser hair removal following forehead flap for nasal reconstruction. Laser Med Sci 2020;35(7). https://doi.org/10.1007/s10103-020-02965-9.

38. Quatela VC, Sherris DA, Rounds MF. Esthetic refinements in forehead flap nasal reconstruction. Arch Otolaryngol Head Neck Surg 1995;121(10):1106–13.

39. Austin GK, Shockley WW. Reconstruction of nasal defects: contemporary approaches. Curr Opin Otolaryngol Head Neck Surg 2016;24(5):453–60.

40. Brightman LA, Brauer JA, Anolik R, et al. Reduction of thickened flap using fractional carbon dioxide laser. Laser Surg Med 2011;43(9):873–4.

41. Rohrich RJ, Griffin JR, Ansari M, et al. Nasal reconstruction–beyond aesthetic subunits: a 15-year review of 1334 cases. Plast Reconstr Surg 2004; 114(6):1405–16. discussion 1417-1419.

42. Veldhuizen IJ, Lee EH, Kurtansky NR, et al. To see or not to see: Impact of viewing facial skin cancer defects prior to reconstruction. Arch Dermatol Res 2021;313(10):847–53.

# Nasal Reconstruction of Large Defects Without a Forehead Flap

John L. Frodel Jr, MD

## KEYWORDS

• Nasal reconstruction • Nasal defect • Nasal deformity • Nasal flaps

## KEY POINTS

• Forehead flaps are a mainstay of large nasal defect reconstruction, yet some clinical scenarios are best treated with less elaborate options.
• Cheek advancement flaps may sometimes be an option for defects of the nasal sidewall or dorsum.
• A combination of local flaps plus skin grafts can be useful on occasion, even for large nasal defects.

## INTRODUCTION

The facial plastic surgeon continues to commonly be presented with challenging defects of the nose, particularly after skin cancer resection. Perhaps some of the most challenging defects are those of an intermediate size, when the surgeon has to decide whether the inherent morbidity of a forehead flap is without question required for normal successful reconstruction. Compounding this issue is the occasional patient who limits reconstructive options due to comorbid health concerns or even unusual concerns such as a very short vertical height of the forehead with an anterior hairline which may limit the ability to use a forehead flap.

Historically, alternative options of interest include the Tagliacozzi multiple-staged marching forearm flap, microvascular free flaps, the Converse scalping flap, and Washio flap, as well as other techniques.[1,2] These will not be reviewed other than to mention them here as they are not commonly used in modern reconstructive surgery.

In this discussion, the author will review alternative options to forehead flaps for reconstructing medium to large nasal skin defects. To be clear, in this author's opinion, defects larger than 2 cm in the nasal tip and columellar region, if full-thickness skin loss, almost always require a forehead flap.

## NASAL DEFECT ANALYSIS

As with any nasal defect, reviewed in many of the other articles in this publication, there are key issues to the analysis of the defect that should always be considered. These include, along with other issues, analysis of the subunits of the nasal skin that are involved, consideration of blood supply, skin thickness issues, structural integrity of the tissues deep to the skin, and whether there is integrity to the internal nasal lining.[2] Without adequate internal lining of the vascularized nature and restructuring of the proper shapes of the various aspects of the nose, the reconstructive outcomes both esthetically and functionally can be compromised.[3] All of these issues will have an impact on the selection of what the reconstructive options are for particular defects of the nose. As each of these important reconstructive considerations will be reviewed in other articles in this publication, they will not be reviewed in detail here.

## NON-FOREHEAD FLAPS FOR NASAL RECONSTRUCTION

This article will specifically review the following for reconstruction of midsized to large-sized nasal defects: primary closure, full-thickness skin grafts,

Guthrie Medical Group, Guthrie Ithaca City Harbor, Otolaryngology, Facial Plastic Surgery, 720 Willow Avenue, Ithaca, NY 14850, USA
E-mail address: John.Frodel@guthrie.org

Facial Plast Surg Clin N Am 32 (2024) 221–227
https://doi.org/10.1016/j.fsc.2024.01.008

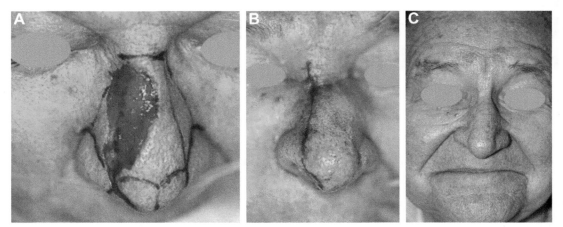

**Fig. 1.** (*A*) Nasal defect after Mohs excision of a lentigo maligna melanoma. (*B*) Intraoperative closure after wide undermining. (*C*) 4-month postoperative result.

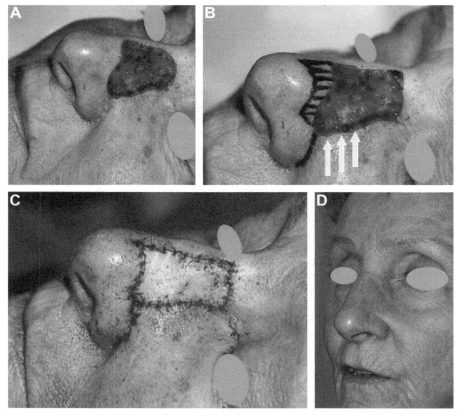

**Fig. 2.** (*A*) Superficial defect after Mohs excision of a basal cell carcinoma involving the lateral dorsal subunit and sidewall subunit of the nose. (*B*) Limited additional incisions were made to allow for the advancement of lateral sidewall and cheek skin as well as dorsal subunits skin to create an isolated sidewall defect. (*C*) After placement of a nasolabial full-thickness skin graft to the sidewall unit. (*D*) 7-month postoperative result.

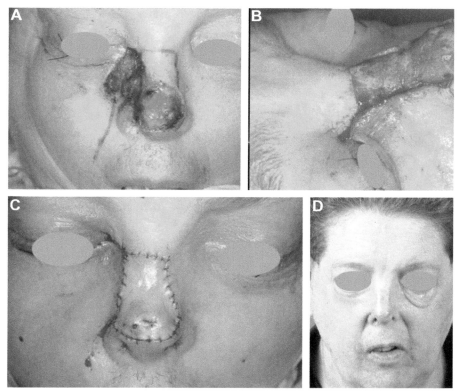

**Fig. 3.** (*A*) Large cutaneous defect of the nasal tip, lower dorsal, right sidewall, and medial cheek subunits after Mohs excision of a lentigo maligna melanoma. (*B*) Medial cheek advancement to create an isolated dorsal and tip subunit defect with good underlying soft tissue bed. (*C*) Full-thickness skin graft placement from the preauricular donor site. (*D*) 6-month postoperative result.

cheek advancement flaps, and nasolabial (melolabial) staged flaps.

### Primary Closure

On somewhat rare occasions, a large defect will present that, after extensive undermining, can be primarily closed.[4,5] **Fig. 1**A shows a patient with a large vertical defect involving the dorsal and sidewall subunits as well as the junction between the tip and right alar subunit. The patient was counseled that a forehead flap may be required and the subunits were marked as well as the forehead flap. However, upon wide undermining, a primary closure that almost perfectly fit into esthetic unit functions was accomplished with a more than satisfactory result (**Fig. 1**B, C). As adjacent tissue is always the best match, particularly when there is some laxity of skin, one should always begin the procedure by widely undermining. This will often facilitate the reconstruction by making the defect smaller or, in some cases, even allow for the closure of the defect without the need for further extensive incisions. This approach works best within the more mobile nasal subunits

of the dorsum, sidewall, glabella, and supratip. There is typically not much ability to undermine the fixed skin subunits of the ala, tip, columella, or soft tissue facets.

### Skin Grafts

While it is not common, there will be an occasion where the skin defect is of a more superficial nature and where there is adequate vascularized soft tissue bed which might accept a skin graft. Usually such skin grafts will be full thickness in nature. Skin texture and color match are important in these cases, so donor site selection is always important. Particularly in an older patient with sun damage in the face, the author has found that harvest of a skin graft from the nasolabial crease region is optimal, with a second choice being preauricular donor skin, and lastly supraclavicular skin donor sites.

With the complexity of subunits being considered, the author has found that even when deciding to use a full-thickness skin graft, there is almost always be some advancement or rotational advancement of some surrounding tissue

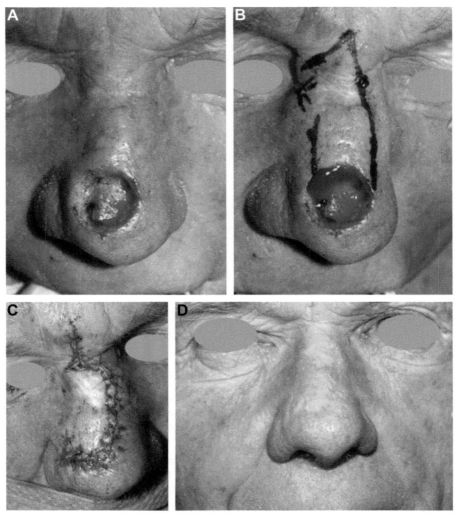

**Fig. 4.** (*A*) Lower central dorsal cutaneous defect after Mohs excision of a basal cell carcinoma. (*B*) Design of a dorsal nasal advancement flap. (*C*) Closure using the dorsal nasal advancement flap. Note some vertical elevation of the tip. (*D*) 3-month postoperative result.

to close subunits adjacent to the subunits that will be reconstructed with a full-thickness skin graft. **Fig. 2** demonstrates this combination in a woman with a basal cell carcinoma who, after Mohs resection, maintained healthy residual underlying tissue bed but with a nasal defect involving both the dorsal and lower lateral sidewall subunits. Advancement of dorsal nasal skin as well as medial cheek skin was then performed to create an isolated left sidewall subunit, which was then reconstructed with a full-thickness skin graft harvested from the right nasolabial crease. **Fig. 3** demonstrates a large defect involving the tip, lower half of the dorsal subunit, all of the lateral sidewall subunit, and extending onto the right cheek after Mohs excision of a lentigo melanoma. A medial

cheek advancement flap was performed to reconstruct the entire right sidewall subunit, then a large preauricular skin graft was used to reconstruct the remaining dorsal and tip subunits.

## Dorsal Nasal or Reiger Advancement Flaps

This flap is often touted for reconstruction of larger tip and lower dorsal subunit skin defects.[6] The author has found it to be useful in a very a limited type of defect, that being the 1.0 to 2.0 cm superior tip and lower dorsal defects. **Fig. 4** shows such a defect where this flap was utilized. One should be aware that the dynamics of the flap will rotate the tip due to tension.[1] Accordingly, the ideal patient is one with a longer perhaps even ptotic

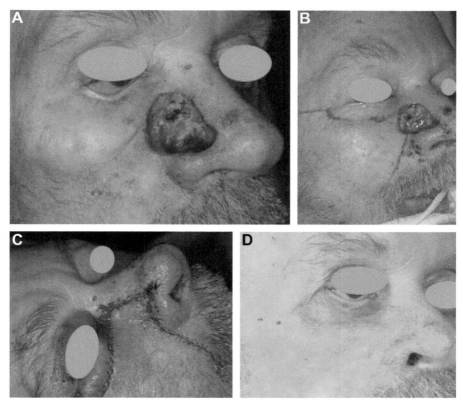

**Fig. 5.** (*A*) Right lateral sidewall defect extending onto the cheek after Mohs excision of a basal cell carcinoma. Note the pre-existing lower eyelid retraction. (*B*) The procedure was begun with lower lid tightening and elevation including a tarsal strip procedure. An incision was made low at the junction between the lower eyelid and the cheek subunit extended into the temple. This allowed for not only horizontal advancement but additional vertical tissue advancement into the lower eyelid to support the eyelid. (*C*) Flaps advanced and eyelid tightened. (*D*) 6-month postoperative result, noting improved lower eyelid position and adequate reconstructive result.

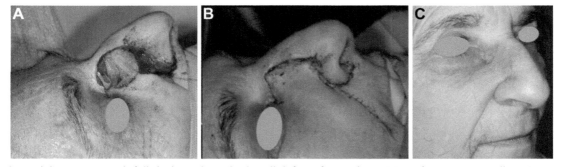

**Fig. 6.** (*A*) A patient with full-thickness lateral sidewall defect after Mohs excision of a squamous cell carcinoma including intranasal involvement. The Mohs excision was supplemented with a left alatomy. (*B*) As structural support is felt to be less important and the intention was to create as little morbidity as possible, the defect was solely reconstructed with a thick cheek advancement flap without reconstruction of the internal lining or structural support. (*C*) 4-month postoperative result.

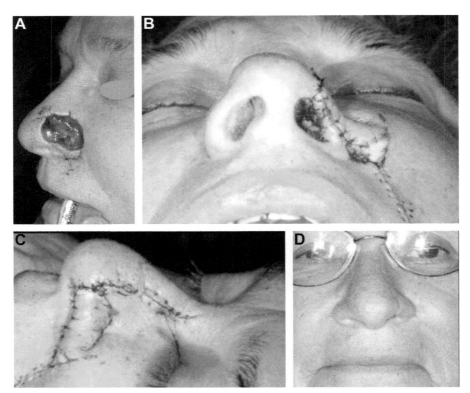

**Fig. 7.** (*A*) A large alar and lower sidewall defect after Mohs excision of a basal cell carcinoma. (*B, C*). Reconstruction using a vertical advancement flap to close the side wall unit defect, followed by a two-stage nasolabial interpolated flap reconstruction of the ala. (*D*) 4-month postoperative result.

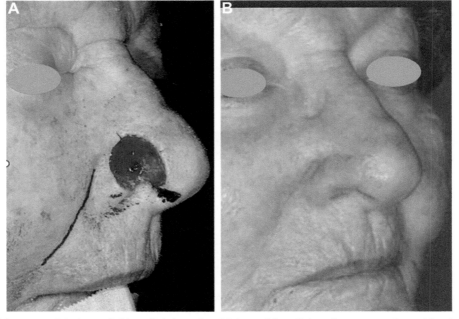

**Fig. 8.** (*A*) Large partial alar and sidewall defect after Mohs excision. Sidewall reconstruction with advancement flap then isolated alar reconstruction with 2-stage nasolabial flap including cartilage batten grafting. (*B*) 3-month postoperative results.

nose who can withstand some tip rotation.[3] When the defect extends further onto the tip, the author finds that this flap is commonly unable to reach the distal end of the defect.

### Cheek Advancement Flaps

Larger total sidewall subunit defects including impingement onto the dorsal subunit might lead one to consider the use of a forehead flap. The author has found that many of these can be reconstructed with large cheek rotation-advancement flaps.[7] Counseling is very important on such cases as, on occasion, the incisions can be extensive along the nasolabial crease as well as extensively into the lower eyelid/cheek junction, and sometimes into the temple region. The latter is particularly important in light of the increased risk of lower eyelid retraction and this should always be considered.

**Fig. 5** shows a man after Mohs excision of a basal cell carcinoma. The defect involves the lateral sidewall subunit and extends onto the cheek, but notice that there is already preoperative retraction of the lower eyelid (likely from previous surgery for senile lid changes). Accordingly, the lower eyelid was prophylactically tightened prior to incisions at the lower eyelid-cheek subunit junction. The incision was intentionally curved upwards to the temporal region so as to allow rotation and advancement not only to reconstruct the nasal defect but also to add vertical tissue augmentation to the lower eyelid for support.

**Fig. 6** shows a full-thickness defect of the sidewall after excision of a squamous cell carcinoma. This was a frail older woman and the decision was to proceed with a limited procedure. No lining or actual support was added as it felt that internal scarring would not impact the final result.

### NasoLabial Flaps

While nasolabial flaps are thought of as a mainstay for alar cutaneous reconstruction, defects that include the ala and surrounding structures can often be reconstructed with a combination of a 2-stage nasolabial flap along with rotation advancement flaps to create an isolated alar defect.[3] Of course, it is important to consider structural reconstruction as well as lining reconstruction needs when the defect is more than just superficial.[2] **Fig. 7** demonstrates a large defect of the ala and lower sidewall unit reconstructed with a vertical advancement flap to close the sidewall defect, followed by 2-stage nasolabial flap, including cartilage batten grafting.

**Fig. 8** demonstrates a similar concept of an advancement flap for the reconstruction of the sidewall unit and nasolabial flap for the reconstruction of the alar subunit.

### SUMMARY

While the multiple-stage paramedian forehead flap remains the mainstay for larger defects of the nose, other options can be utilized in certain types of defects for the nose. These are particularly important when staged procedures create more of a problem with morbidity that can be required when using multiple staged forehead flaps.

### CLINICS CARE POINTS

- Think of options besides forehead flaps, particularly for lateral nasal defects.
- Occasionally, full-thickness skin grafts may be an option for thin or optimally located defects.
- Extended cheek-advancement or large local nasal flaps may be useful even in scenarios most commonly treated with a forehead flap.
- A combination of flaps or skin graft with flap may occasionally be an option.
- Various patient factors, medical comorbidities, or defect characteristics may favor reconstruction with techniques other than a forehead flap.

### DISCLOSURE

The authors have nothing to disclose.

### REFERENCES

1. Baker SR. Reconstruction of the Nose. In: Baker SR, editor. "Local flaps in facial reconstruction". Elsevier; 2022.
2. Burget FJ, Menick FJ. Aesthetic reconstruction of the nose. 2nd edition. St. Louis: Mosby; 1993.
3. Baker SR, editor. Principles of nasal reconstruction. 2nd edition. New York: Springer; 2011.
4. Neill B, Rickstrew J, Tolkachjov. Reconstructing the glabella and nasal root. J Drugs Dermatol JDD 2022; 21:983–8.
5. Wesley NO, Yu SS, Grekin RC, et al. Primary linear closure for large defects of the nasal supratip. Dermatol Surg 2008;34:380–4.
6. Eren E, Beden V. Beyond Rieger's original indication; the dorsal nasal flap revisited. J Cranio-Maxillo-Fac Surg 2014;42:412–6.
7. Haugen T, Frodel JL. Reconstruction of complex nasal dorsal and sidewall defects: is the nasal sidewall subunit necessary. Arch Facial Plast Surg 2011; 13:343–6.

# Nasal Lining Reconstruction with Locoregional Flaps

Alexander E. Graf, MD[a], Lee Kaplowitz, MD[b], Sydney C. Butts, MD[a],*

## KEYWORDS

- Full-thickness nasal defect • Nasal lining flaps • Bipedicle vestibular advancement flap
- Septal mucoperichondrial flap • Inferior turbinate flap • Pericranial flap

## KEY POINTS

- Flaps developed from nasal sources for lining can usually line one or a maximum of 2 subunits. Extensive lining deficits will require multiple local flaps used in combination or an extranasal flap for lining.
- Patients should be thoroughly counseled about the donor site morbidity associated with the development of certain intranasal lining flaps, which can result in prolonged aftercare for the management of symptoms associated with septal perforation, crusting, and rhinorrhea.
- Endoscopic assistance is valuable in elevating intranasal lining flaps-providing magnified visualization for raising of flaps, which may require retrograde dissection of tissues.
- Intranasal flap harvesting requires delicate tissue handling and proper instrumentation. Rhinoplasty instruments along with other specialized nasal instruments that may be available on a sinus set are important to ensure safe flap harvest.

 Video content accompanies this article at http://www.facialplastic.theclinics.com

## INTRODUCTION

The leading causes of soft tissue loses of the nose include traumatic causes and postoncologic defects after excision of melanoma or nonmelanoma skin cancers. The nose is the most common location for skin cancers to develop on the face.[1,2] Numerous considerations are involved in the nasal reconstructive plan to restore form and function. The 3 layers of the nose—external cover, osseocartilaginous support, and lining—all contribute to form and function in important ways. This article will focus on the importance of replacing nasal lining. The nasal lining should be thought of as the foundation for nasal reconstruction. Intact nasal lining is a barrier between the nasal airway (and therefore nasal secretions) and nasal soft tissues.

When the lining is missing and not replaced, the raw surface will heal by secondary intention causing contracture and narrowing of the airway. Vascularized lining is also critical for supporting cartilage or bone grafts used to replace the nasal framework.

## ANATOMY

Sources of tissue to replace nasal lining developed from intranasal soft tissue will consist of either skin or mucosa. The nasal vestibule is lined by hair-bearing skin. At the mucocutaneous junction, also called the limen nasi, the nasal skin transitions to respiratory mucosa.[3,4] Medially, this transition occurs at the junction of the membranous septum and the caudal cartilaginous septum and laterally

[a] Department of Otolaryngology, SUNY Downstate Health Sciences University, 450 Clarkson Avenue, Brooklyn, NY 11203, USA; [b] Division of Otolaryngology, Department of Surgery, Maimonides Medical Center, 4802 Tenth Avenue, Brooklyn, NY 11219, USA
* Corresponding author.
E-mail address: Sydney.butts@downstate.edu

Facial Plast Surg Clin N Am 32 (2024) 229–237
https://doi.org/10.1016/j.fsc.2024.01.003
1064-7406/24/© 2024 Elsevier Inc. All rights reserved.

at approximately the scroll area where the lateral crus of the lower lateral cartilage and the caudal upper lateral cartilage meet.[5] Understanding the nature of the available donor tissues (skin or mucosa) and their location determines characteristics of the flap that can be harvested including pliability, quantity, reach, and mucous secretion. Given the robust blood supply of the nose, local intranasal flaps are very reliable. The flaps that will be described in this article receive their blood supply from branches of the superior labial artery, angular artery, or ethmoid arteries (**Fig. 1**). The flaps developed from extranasal donor sites are also based on branches of the facial/angular artery system, with the exception of the pericranial flap, which is supplied by the supratrochlear artery.

## INTERNAL NASAL LINING FLAPS
### Bipedicled Vestibular Advancement

The bipedicled vestibular advancement flap, first described by Burget and Menick in 1986 and later popularized by Shan Baker in 1998, is ideally suited for the reconstruction of lining defects of the nasal ala and adjacent hemitip up to 1.5 cm in height.[6–8] The vestibular skin is mobilized with an extended

intercartilaginous incision at the junction of the skin and nasal mucosa made from the dome of the lower lateral cartilage medially extending to the nasal floor laterally. Additional flap mobilization can be achieved by extending the medial incision toward the membranous septum. The flap is dissected from the overlying cartilage, mobilized caudally, and inset along the inferior edge of the defect. The flap must be fixed to the reconstructed cartilaginous framework, to prevent alar retraction. Depending on the extent of caudal mobilization, the raw area left intranasally can either be closed primarily, covered with a full thickness skin graft or with a caudally based septal mucosal flap.[9]

The case in **Fig. 2** shows a patient following Mohs excision of a basal cell carcinoma of the nose resulting in a 1 cm × 5 mm full thickness defect of the left nostril rim involving the junction of the alar and tip subunits (see **Fig. 2**). A bipedicled vestibular advancement flap was developed from the adjacent vestibular skin for lining. Using endoscopic assistance, an incision was made parallel to the free edge of the defect in the area of the junction of the superior vestibular skin and the intranasal mucosa, leaving the flap anchored medially and laterally (Video 1) This

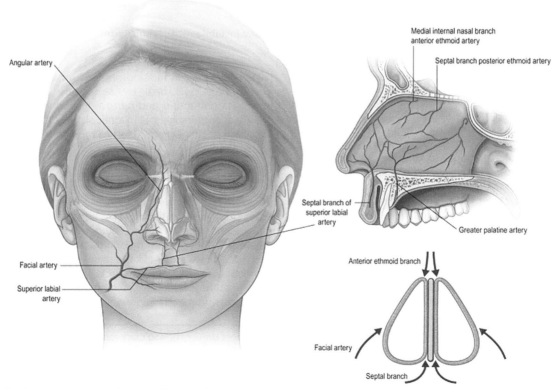

**Fig. 1.** Blood supply to intranasal mucosal used for lining flaps. (Joseph E. Losee, Peter C. Neligan, Plastic Surgery: Volume 3: Craniofacial, Head and Neck Surgery and Pediatric Plastic Surgery, 3rd edition, Saunders, 2012.)

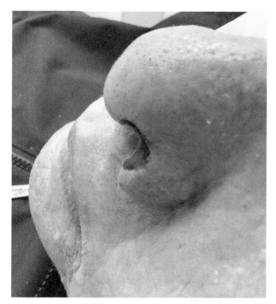

**Fig. 2.** A full-thickness defect of the left nostril rim involving the junction of the anterior ala and tip subunit.

dissection allowed inferior movement of the flap to the nostril rim. The defect created by flap mobilization was narrow and closed primarily. An auricular cartilage graft was placed at the rim and sutured to the vestibular lining flap with absorbable sutures (**Fig. 3**). A superiorly based melolabial flap was rotated for cover (**Fig. 4**) and divided and inset 3 weeks later (**Fig. 5**).

Advantages of this flap are the use of thin, physiologically similar tissue that is inset in one stage. The main disadvantage is inability to reconstruct defects larger than the height of the ala. The raw donor area must be covered to prevent contracture in the area of the scroll.

### Septal Flaps

Variations of septal flaps have been used for decades for reconstruction of nasal lining. Despite historical and widespread use, Burget and Menick in 1989 were the first to describe the blood supply of the inferior pedicle to the caudal septum: the septal branch of the superior labial artery from the facial artery[10] (see **Fig. 1**). As long as the pedicle is maintained, unilateral or bilateral septal mucoperichondrial flaps can be harvested, and composite flaps with cartilage attached can also be developed. Branches of the ethmoid arteries support the development of dorsally based septal flaps.

### Septal mucoperichondrial flap

Lining defects of the nasal alar subunit can be reconstructed using a caudally based septal

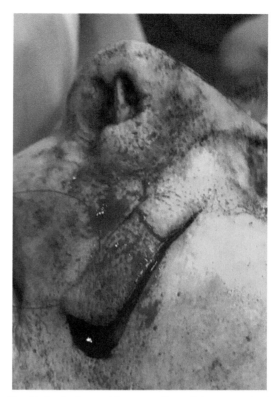

**Fig. 3.** Auricular cartilage graft used to reconstruct alar rim framework after rotation of a bipedicled vestibular flap.

mucoperichondrial flap ipsilateral to the defect (**Fig. 6**). If the flap is designed up to its maximal dimensions, it can extend to line an alar defect that also involves the hemitip and/or part of the adjacent nasal sidewall. The septal branch of the superior labial artery provides sufficient blood supply to harvest a septal flap that spans the height of the

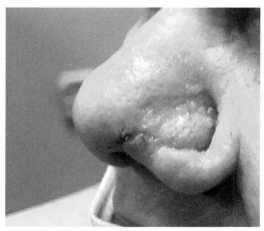

**Fig. 4.** Inset of the melolabial flap used for coverage of the alar rim defect.

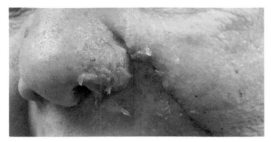

**Fig. 5.** Division of melolabial flap pedicle used for coverage of alar rim defect.

septum and extends posteriorly to beyond the bony-cartilaginous junction with dimensions up to 4 cm in length and 2.5 cm in width possible. An incision along the dorsal septal mucosa roughly 1 cm inferior to the roof of the nose is made extending posteriorly beyond the location of the bony-cartilaginous junction. This incision is connected to a posterior vertical incision that is brought to the floor of the nose. The final incision is made parallel to the dorsal nasal incision and ends posterior to the anterior nasal spine (see **Fig. 6**, Video 2). The horizontal incisions should not involve mucosa of the caudal septum. Once the flap incisions are complete, the flap is elevated retrograde toward the vestibule and transposed to the location of the new ala (**Fig. 7**). The flap is anchored in place to the edges of the defect with absorbable sutures. Where the flap curves and meets the nasal sidewall, it is suspended to the free edge to close off the connection between the nasal airway and the reconstructed area.

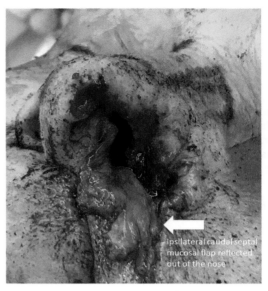

Ipsilateral caudal septal mucosal flap reflected out of the nose

**Fig. 7.** Multisubunit left nasal defect involving the ala, sidewall, and hemitip. Caudal septal mucosal flap harvest for lining, reflected out of the nose in preparation for inset.

Cartilage grafts are placed over the lining flap, which is suspended to the undersurface of the grafts with absorbable sutures (**Fig. 8**). This flap will obstruct the nasal vestibule and require detachment at a second stage from the pedicle, which can be performed at the same time as the division and inset of the regional flap used for external cover.

For middle vault coverage, a contralateral septal flap based dorsally on the ethmoid arteries is used. In order to accomplish this, a septal perforation must be created, removing the quadrangular cartilage to allow the flap to be transposed to the other

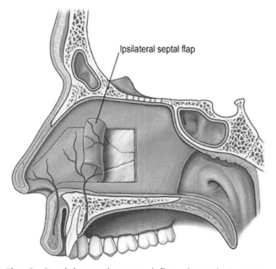

Ipsilateral septal flap

**Fig. 6.** Caudal septal mucosal flap. (Joseph E. Losee, Peter C. Neligan, Plastic Surgery: Volume 3: Craniofacial, Head and Neck Surgery and Pediatric Plastic Surgery, 3rd edition, Saunders, 2012.)

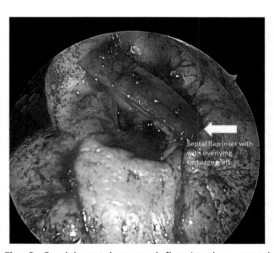

Septal flap inset with with overlying cartilage graft

**Fig. 8.** Caudal septal mucosal flap in place, septal cartilage graft sutured to flap.

side of the nasal cavity. The standard dorsal strut of 1.2 to 1.5 cm must be maintained.[9] These flaps can be combined to line defects that involve numerous nasal subunits. The ipsilateral caudal septal flap can be combined with the contralateral dorsal septal flap to reconstruct lining defects of the lower two-thirds of the nasal vault (alar, sidewall, and hemitip defects). Bilateral caudal septal mucosal flaps can be developed and combined to replace lining of a full thickness nasal tip defect. Underlying septal cartilage is harvested and used for grafting, leaving a permanent septal perforation.

### Septal composite chondromucosal flap

To reconstruct nasal lining and provide structural tip support, a septal chondromucosal flap can be harvested based on bilateral septal artery branches. This flap is ideal for the reconstruction of central, full thickness defects involving the tip.[9] In this procedure, the residual septum is harvested as a flap and pivoted 90° anteriorly to reconstruct the caudal strut (**Fig. 9**).

### Inferior Turbinate Mucoperichondrial Flap

The inferior turbinate mucoperichondrial flap is a viable option to restore lining for the ala or caudal

sidewall.[11] The flap is hinged anteriorly and transposed by first separating the bony attachment of the turbinate from the nasal sidewall and then delivering the turbinate, attached at the head, anteriorly out of the nose. The bone is dissected away from the mucoperiosteum and the flap inset. Up to 5 cm² of mucosal surface area can be harvested.[11]

Advantages of this flap are the preservation of the septum and its robust blood supply. If the lining defect extends to the nasal tip, the flap may partially obstruct the nasal airway, requiring transection of the base of the flap at a second stage.[12] In contrast to the bipedicled vestibular flap used for alar lining reconstruction, this flap replaces skin with mucosa. Mucous secreting tissue is placed at the alar margin rather than skin, which can result in bothersome rhinorrhea for the patient.

### HINGE-FLAP (TURN-IN)

The cutaneous hinge or "turn-in" flap (**Fig. 10**) uses surrounding skin that has healed to the edges of the defect, allowing skin to be developed as short flaps supplied by the subcutaneous blood supply.[13] These flaps cannot be used to reconstruct

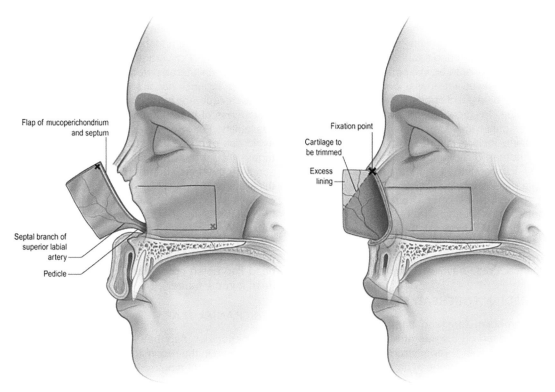

**Fig. 9.** Reconstruction of dorsal cartilaginous defect with septal pivot flap. (Joseph E. Losee, Peter C. Neligan, Plastic Surgery: Volume 3: Craniofacial, Head and Neck Surgery and Pediatric Plastic Surgery, 3rd edition, Saunders, 2012.)

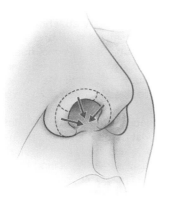 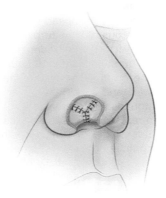

**Fig. 10.** Turn-in hinge flaps for lining. (Joseph E. Losee, Peter C. Neligan, Plastic Surgery: Volume 3: Craniofacial, Head and Neck Surgery and Pediatric Plastic Surgery, 3rd edition, Saunders, 2012.)

an acute nasal lining defect and are used in cases performed in a delayed fashion. The vascularity of these flaps is less robust than others previously described and the maximal recommended flap length should not exceed 1.5 cm. The skin is incised the length that is needed to reach the opposite edge of the defect and "turned-in" 180° with the skin facing the nasal airway. The design of the flaps depends on the size and location of the defect and may be designed as one flap or several depending on the shape of the defect (see **Fig. 10**).

This flap avoids the creation of an additional donor site. The harvested skin should not extend beyond the boundaries of the involved nasal subunit requiring lining unless that skin will be replaced by the covering flap.[14] If there are several lining options considered in a pediatric case, a turn in flap that leaves intranasal donor sites undisturbed may be a good choice that avoids potential scar tissue in growth centers of the nose.[9] Possible challenges encountered when using hinge flaps include stiffness of the tissues and bulk. Another disadvantage of this flap is the inability to reconstruct a larger defect involving multiple nasal subunits because the length of the flaps must be shorter than the previously described flaps that have more robust vascularity. Finally, because external nasal skin with solar damage in the region of the resected skin cancer will be transposed intransally, a new or recurrent skin cancer could develop within the nasal cavity.

## PARAMEDIAN FOREHEAD FLAP

The paramedian forehead flap, an interpolated, axial flap based on the supratrochlear artery, can be used for lining reconstruction as well as external cover. The forehead flap can be designed with a superior extension designed to replace the lining defect by folding the skin of the flap intranasally to replace the missing lining. Extension into the hair-bearing scalp is appropriate if the extension will be used for lining of an alar defect, which was previously lined with hair-bearing skin. After harvest, the extension is folded over the alar rim and sutured to residual lining.[15] Cartilage framework can be placed between the layers of the forehead flap at an intermediate stage, before final division of the pedicle.

The paramedian forehead flap can be used exclusively for lining by rotating it with the skin side facing the nasal airway.[16] In this approach, a through and through skin incision is made over the lateral nasal side wall to tunnel the flap into position so it may be secured to the residual nasal lining. Paired paramedian forehead flaps have been described for simultaneous reconstruction of nasal lining and coverage. This technique is well suited for unilateral defects greater than 2 cm involving superior nasal subunits. Advantages of this technique are familiarity and ease of harvest, robustness of blood supply, and generous tissue availability. For large defects, use of this flap can avoid use of a microvascular free flap. Disadvantages are intranasal bulk and multiple external scars on the nose and forehead. It is important to think about the possibility of recurrent/future skin cancers in patients if bilateral paramedian forehead flaps are to be used in one reconstructive case. While elevating another forehead flap at the site of a prior harvest might be possible, difficulties may be encountered, eliminating the forehead flap as an option for the patient who might need it in the future.

## PERICRANIAL FLAP

The pericranial flap has been reliably used for many years in the reconstruction of skull base defects, for frontal sinus obliteration, and for scalp reconstruction. Its use in reconstructing intranasal lining for nasal defects is a relatively recent application. Sertel and colleagues demonstrated the feasibility of this flap for nasal reconstruction including the ability to harvest a flap up to 70 mm in length and should be based on the supraorbital artery to ensure vascularity of a flap of that length.[17]

A case series by Lewis and colleagues demonstrated the utility of this flap.[18] Of the 18 patients for whom the pericranial flap was harvested for lining, no patients had immediate postoperative complications. Three of the patients who had reconstructive failure did so after radiation therapy. Other reported complications were nasal stenosis and fistula.

The use of the pericranial flap for nasal lining reconstruction is well suited for midvault defects serving as the base for cartilage or bone grafts. Often this flap is paired with a paramedian forehead flap, which allows harvesting via the same incision site.

A full thickness defect of the nasal dorsum and left nasal sidewall following trauma shown in **Fig. 11** demonstrates how the pericranial flap can be used. The specific patient factors that lead to this decision were the size of the defect, accessibility through the planned paramedian incision, and the lack of septal tissue as a donor site for lining.

## MELOLABIAL FLAP

The melolabial cheek flap has been a workhorse flap for nasal reconstruction for centuries.[19] A single-staged, subcutaneous flap taken from the nasolabial fold for nasal lining reconstruction was first described in 1953 by Roberto Farina in a patient with nasal tip collapse secondary to leprosy.[20] In 1967, Pers first described use of a similar, extended melolabial flap turned in on itself to reconstruct both the nasal lining and skin coverage.[19] This flap is supplied by cutaneous perforators of the angular arteries.

Baker advocates for designing the interpolated cheek flap such that the center of the flap lies 1 cm above the horizontal plane of the oral commissure with the medial border lying on the nasolabial fold.[21] Using similar flap design, Griffin and colleagues first described the use of the melolabial flap in a 2-staged approach for lining reconstruction in 2013. The flap is raised in an inferior to superior direction, then turned over, and inset into the defect.[22]

Advantages of using this flap are ability to place the scar in the melo-labial crease, ability to harvest a large amount of new lining, ease of harvest, and robustness of flap blood supply.[22,23] Disadvantages are possibly creating facial asymmetry and bulk, which make it less frequently used at present.

## FACIAL ARTERY BASED MUCOSAL AND MUSCULOMUCOSAL FLAP

Variations of axial flaps based on the facial artery are well-established options for nasal lining reconstruction.[24] The facial artery musculomucosal (FAMM) flap popularized by Pribaz and colleagues in 1991 includes buccal mucosa, submucosa, and buccinator muscle.[25] Using an oblique orientation extending from the retromolar trigone to the upper buccal mucosa with either an inferiorly or superiorly based pedicle, a 1.5 to 2 cm × 8 to 9 cm flap can be harvested. Duffy, Rossi, and Pribaz, described the use of bilateral FAMM flaps for reconstruction of the nasal lining in a patient with a saddle nose deformity secondary to Wegener granulomatosis.[26] After harvest, the flap is

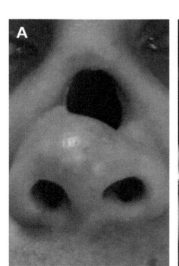
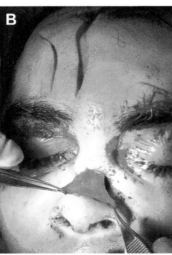

**Fig. 11.** (*A*) A full-thickness defect of nasal dorsum and left nasal sidewall. (*B*) Pericranial flap tunneled deep to the skin surrounding the defect. Right paramedian forehead flap has been incised.

tunneled through the alar base to reconstruct the lining.[9] FAMM flaps for lining reconstruction are typically reserved for cases in which there is limited local tissue availability.[27] This flap is particularly useful for middle third lining reconstruction with extensive surrounding tissue loss.[9] The donor site defect can be closed primarily with minimal donor site morbidity. Advantages of this flap include ease of harvest, lack of external scars, and robustness of flap blood supply. A disadvantage of the FAMM flap is excessive tissue bulk, which can reduce nasal airway airflow and may require a later debulking procedure.

## DISCUSSION

Although not the visible part of the reconstruction, lining restoration is integral to successful outcomes in treating full-thickness nasal defects. Regardless of the reconstructive plan for the external aspect of the nasal defect, a vascularized internal lining is vital to support the grafts and flaps that will be used. The success of the flaps described depends on patient factors and optimal donor site conditions. The timing and options for flaps will differ based on whether reconstruction is required for trauma or reconstruction after skin cancer or other causes. Caution must be exercised in harvesting a flap for lining from an area that has been previously operated on, where there has been prior significant trauma or if the tissues have been exposed to radiation. Patient factors including current or recent tobacco use or any history of intranasal drug use significantly increase the risk of flap failure.

## SUMMARY

Internal lining reconstruction is the foundation on which the framework and external reconstruction are built. Selecting the appropriate flap, understanding its applications and its blood supply are paramount for surgical planning.

## CLINICS CARE POINTS

- Complications associated with the use of flaps to restore lining should be low as long as the vascular supply underlying each unique flap design is respected. Some of the incisions are different from incisions typically used in septal surgery or rhinoplasty, which must be remembered to avoid disrupting the blood supply on which the flap is pedicled.
- Postoperative evaluation of intranasal donor sites may require in-office nasal endoscopy to assess any healing problems including sites of granulation tissue formation, intranasal synechiae, crusting, and septal perforation.

## DISCLOSURE

None of the authors have any disclosures.

## SUPPLEMENTARY DATA

Supplementary data related to this article can be found online at https://doi.org/10.1016/j.fsc.2024.01.003.

## REFERENCES

1. Fijałkowska M, Koziej M, Antoszewski B. Detailed head localization and incidence of skin cancers. Sci Rep 2021;11(1):12391.
2. National Comprehensive Cancer Network. Squamous Cell Skin Cancer (Version 1.2023). https://www.nccn.org/professionals/physician_gls/pdf/squamous.pdf. Accessed October 18, 2023.
3. Bussu F, Tagliaferri L, Piras A, et al. Multidisciplinary approach to nose vestibule malignancies: setting new standards. Acta Otorhinolaryngol Ital 2021;41(Suppl.1):S158–65.
4. Kim SJ, Byun SW, Lee SS. Various tumors in the nasal vestibule. Int J Clin Exp Pathol 2013;6(12):2713–8.
5. Patel RG. Nasal Anatomy and Function. Facial Plast Surg 2017;33(1):3–8.
6. Burget GC, Menick FJ. Nasal reconstruction: seeking a fourth dimension. Plast Reconstr Surg 1986;78(2):145–57.
7. Baker SR. Nasal lining flaps in contemporary reconstructive rhinoplasty. Facial Plast Surg 1998;14(2):133–44.
8. Baker SR. Flap classification and design. In: Baker SR, editor. Local flaps in facial reconstruction. 3rd edition. Philadelphia, PA: Elsevier/Saunders; 2014. p. 71–107.
9. Menick FJ. Nasal reconstruction: Art and practice. New York, NY: Elsevier; 2008.
10. Burget GC, Menick FJ. Nasal support and lining: the marriage of beauty and blood supply. Plast Reconstr Surg 1989;84(2):189–202.
11. Murakami CS, Kriet JD, Ierokomos AP. Nasal reconstruction using the inferior turbinate mucosal flap. Arch Facial Plast Surg 1999;1(2):97–100.
12. Baker SR. Reconstruction of the nose. In: Baker SR, editor. Local flaps in facial reconstruction. 3rd edition. Philadelphia, PA: Elsevier/Saunders; 2014. p. 415–80.

13. Park SS, Cook TA, Wang TD. The epithelial 'turn-in' flap in nasal reconstruction. Arch Otolaryngol Head Neck Surg 1995;121(10):1122–7.

14. Ulug BT, Kuran I. Nasal reconstruction based on subunit principle combined with turn-over island nasal skin flap for nasal lining restoration. Ann Plast Surg 2008;61(5):521–6.

15. Menick FJ. A new modified method for nasal lining: the Menick technique for folded lining. J Surg Oncol 2006;94(6):509–14.

16. Parikh S, Futran ND, Most SP. An alternative method for reconstruction of large intranasal lining defects: the Farina method revisited. Arch Facial Plast Surg 2010;12(5):311–4.

17. Sertel S, Pasche P. Pericranial flap for inner lining in nasal reconstruction. Ann Plast Surg 2016;77(4):425–32.

18. Lewis T, Care R, Kuta V, et al. The pericranial flap for inner lining of full-thickness nasal defects: a retrospective cohort study. J Laryngol Otol 2023;137(5):532–6.

19. Pers M. Cheek flaps in partial rhinoplasty: a new variation: the in-and-out flap. Scand J Plast Reconstr Surg 1967;1(1):37–44.

20. Farina R. Nose tip collapse through loss of chondromucous substance (repair of nasal lining). Plast Reconstr Surg 1954;13(2):137–43.

21. Baker SR. Melolabial flaps. In: Baker SR, editor. Local flaps in facial reconstruction. 3rd edition. Philadelphia, PA: Elsevier/Saunders; 2014. p. 231–67.

22. Griffin GR, Chepeha DB, Moyer JS. Interpolated subcutaneous fat pedicle melolabial flap for large nasal lining defects. Laryngoscope 2013;123(2):356–9.

23. Lane JE, Bob Hsia LL, Merritt BG. Reconstruction of large transmural nasal defects with a nasolabial turnover interpolation flap. Dermatol Surg 2020;46(7):899–903.

24. Soutar DS, Elliot D, Rao GS. Buccal mucosal flaps in nasal reconstruction. Br J Plast Surg 1990;43(5):612–6.

25. Pribaz J, Stephens W, Crespo L, et al. A new intraoral flap: facial artery musculomucosal (FAMM) flap. Plast Reconstr Surg 1992;90(3):421–9.

26. Duffy FJ Jr, Rossi RM, Pribaz JJ. Reconstruction of Wegener's nasal deformity using bilateral facial artery musculomucosal flaps. Plast Reconstr Surg 1998;101(5):1330–3.

27. Yen CI, Chang CS, Chen HC, et al. The upper buccal musculomucosal flap for nasal lining and columellar defect reconstruction. J Craniofac Surg 2021;32(5):1850–2.

# Nasal Lining Reconstruction with Prelaminated Forehead Flap

Khashayar Arianpour, MD[a], Patrick J. Byrne, MD, MBA[b],*

## KEYWORDS

• Forehead flap • Prelaminated • Prefabricated • Nasal reconstruction • Nasal lining

## KEY POINTS

- The prelaminated paramedian forehead flap comprises a four-stage technique that allows for the multilaminar composite reconstruction of partial to total nasal defects.
- Prelamination using a split-thickness skin graft confers several advantages to successfully restore the internal nasal lining.
- The result is an abundant, pliable, and vascularized nasal lining with minimal bulk that adequately supports the structural framework.
- Patients must be cautioned that the technique adds a stage, prolongs pedicle takedown, and leaves the primary defect unaddressed during the first stage.

 Video content accompanies this article at http://www.facialplastic.theclinics.com.

## INTRODUCTION

Addressing partial to total nasal defects is a challenging reconstructive endeavor. Its approach is often categorized into 3 tasks: restoring structural support, restoring external cutaneous lining, and restoring internal mucosal lining. Often, the latter task is the limiting factor in achieving a successful reconstruction as obtaining tissue of adequate size and pliability with longstanding stability can be difficult. The prelamination technique uses a staged skin graft to the paramedian forehead flap prior to transfer. This multilaminar composite flap can be transferred as a single unit to reconstruct internal and external nasal defects concomitantly.[1] This article reviews current methods, techniques, and other clinical considerations in the use of the prelaminated forehead flap for nasal lining reconstruction in partial to total nasal defects.

## BACKGROUND

While the external nose has long been recognized as the keystone of facial aesthetics, its internal counterpart, the nasal cavity, serves as a complex physiologic organ that hosts a myriad of functions that cannot be overlooked. A successful reconstructive facial plastic surgeon must restore nasal symmetry while maintaining respiratory function. Importantly, internal nasal stability drives external nasal stability, and as such, achieving the former is crucial to a successful reconstruction.

The nasal vestibule is delineated from the nasal cavity by a mucosal ridge the limen naris. The

[a] Department of Otolaryngology - Head and Neck Surgery, Cleveland Clinic Head and Neck Institute, Cleveland Clinic, A7 Crile, 9500 Euclid Avenue, Cleveland, OH 44195. USA; [b] Section of Facial Plastic and Reconstructive Surgery, Department of Otolaryngology - Head and Neck Surgery, Cleveland Clinic Head and Neck Institute, Cleveland Clinic, A7 Crile, 9500 Euclid Avenue, Cleveland, OH 44195, USA
* Corresponding author. Section of Facial Plastic and Microvascular Surgery, Cleveland Clinic, A7 Crile, 9500 Euclid Avenue, Cleveland, OH 44195.
E-mail address: byrnep@ccf.org

Facial Plast Surg Clin N Am 32 (2024) 239–246
https://doi.org/10.1016/j.fsc.2024.02.001
1064-7406/24/© 2024 Elsevier Inc. All rights reserved.

anterior half of the nasal vestibule is lined by stratified keratinizing squamous epithelium containing vibrissae, which filter air particles. The posterior half, along with the remaining entirety of nasal cavities and paranasal sinuses are lined with pseudostratified ciliated columnar epithelium and mucous-secreting glands, termed the respiratory mucosa. This specialized epithelium functions to humidify and warm inhaled air for respiration and trap debris to expel it via mucociliary clearance toward the nasopharynx. Mucous also serves as an immunologic protective barrier and contains odor-binding proteins that are necessary for olfaction.[2] Lastly, but perhaps most importantly, the nasal cavities act as a conduit for inspiration, and thus their obstruction leads to significant dysfunction and an impact on the quality of life.[3]

Ideally, the reconstructive surgeon would be able to restore all internal nasal functions. However, unfortunately, no single technique can achieve this, and depending on the size and location of the defect, one must prioritize one function over another. In the setting of partial to total nasal defects, maintaining airway patency becomes of utmost importance in reconstruction. If the extirpated respiratory epithelium is not replaced, in an attempt to obliterate the defect, scar contracture will ensue, resulting in nasal obstruction.[4] The contracted healing process may cause the remnant tissue to be either drawn in toward the defect, or, excessive inflammatory tissue deposition may cause a mass effect, ultimately causing narrowing of the nasal passage.[5] Reconstitution of the internal nasal lining does not merely aim to restore physiologic function but also determines the external outcome.[6] Internal nasal contracture from an inadequate lining may lead to structural imbalance resulting in amorphous changes in the external reconstruction.[7] In fact, this is not only limited to the nose. In large defects involving the nasal floor, insufficient coverage can lead to the contracture and displacement of the upper lip, resulting in disfiguring changes. Failure to restore the nasal lining can also lead to graft exposure to nasal contents, placing the structural reconstruction directly at risk for chronic infection and ultimate graft loss.[8]

### The Challenge

Reconstruction of the nasal lining is a particularly challenging endeavor for several reasons.

1. It is difficult to obtain suitable graft material. The ideal graft should be well-vascularized to encourage primary healing, fight infection, and nourish structural grafts to protect them from resorption and extrusion. In other words, vascularity drives internal nasal stability, which in turn

ensures external reconstructive longevity. Although the chosen graft requires robust microcirculation, it must also be thin. If too bulky, the reconstruction will defeat the primary purpose that it sought to serve– airway patency. Moreover, this thin graft must also be pliable enough to conform to the three-dimensional structure of the nasal cavity. The graft must satisfy these low-profile properties yet carry sufficient intrinsic strength to counteract significant forces from tissue contracture.[9]

2. The second challenge is obtaining adequate graft size. Limited graft availability is particularly a barrier in partial to total nasal defects. For example, many defects often require coverage of the nasal floor, columella, and nasal vault. For perspective, coverage of the nasal vault from one alar base to the other (through the nasal tip) requires approximately 8 cm of graft.[8]

3. The final challenge is accessibility. Even with ample amounts of the perfect graft material, the location of the defect makes for poor visualization and surgical access.[4] One must inset a graft endonasally while ensuring appropriate contact with the underlying wound bed for the early perioperative period. Moreover, the graft must be secured without the disruption of the limited remaining native nasal mucosa to preserve its physiologic function.

The approach to nasal lining reconstruction is often determined by the size of the intranasal defect. Earlier in this issue, the use of nasal loco-regional flaps was discussed. Although these flaps provide a vascularized, physiologically active, thin flap, they are unfortunately often too small for use in partial to total nasal defects.[1] To obtain sufficient tissue, other options have been suggested. Free skin grafts were proposed by Menick and colleagues, however, this was soon largely abandoned due to their propensity for contracture and resulting amorphous changes to the external nose.[5] Others propose free tissue transfer with microvascular anastomosis, but, these often require more extensive surgery and result in excess bulk.[10]

As we will see, the prelaminated forehead flap technique overcomes many of these challenges. This technique carries all the advantages of the paramedian forehead flap, the workhorse in partial to total nasal reconstruction, while also allowing both external and internal reconstruction concurrently.

### PRELAMINATION

Flap prelamination refers to the addition of tissue to an existing elevated flap with an established vascular bed without compromising its blood supply. The result is a multilayered flap that can be transferred for complex reconstruction in a staged fashion. Strictly speaking, prelamination must not be confused with prefabrication, which is defined as the implantation of a vascular pedicle into a proposed flap, either via free tissue transfer with microvascular anastomosis or regional transfer, followed by delayed regional or distant transfer. In other words, prefabrication creates a vascularized bed (ie, neovascularization) while prelamination takes advantage of one that already exists.[11]

Prelamination techniques date back to the early 1900s.[7] For example, in 1902, Nelaton described the implantation of cartilaginous grafts beneath a forehead flap prior to rotational transfer.[7,12,13] Pioneer Sir Harold Gilles described several prelamination techniques for facial reconstruction in the 1940s.[14] Much of our current understanding of prelamination principles stems from extensive experience with its utilization in free flap reconstruction for multilayered defects.[7,15,16] Although it is unclear who was the first to describe the modern prelamination technique, it is evident that it is the result of several modifications over the last few decades. Lamination of the forehead flap for nasal reconstruction was initially described in the early 2000s using the pericranial flap (either as a separate or shared pedicle) with intervening cartilaginous grafts.[17,18] Around the same time, Gassner and colleagues introduced the in-situ placement of split-thickness skin graft to the forehead flap followed by staged transfer for the nasal lining.[6] This concept of delayed transfer stemmed from lessons learned by Menick's prior experience noting significant contracture after skin grafting of the forehead flap when used at the time of initial transfer.[9] Gassner and colleagues demonstrated that awaiting contracture to take place prior to transfer leads to improved functional and aesthetic outcomes.[6] In a previous section of this issue, the benefits of staged reconstruction were discussed—the prelamination forehead technique is a case in point.

## PREOPERATIVE ASSESSMENT

As with any preoperative assessment, a detailed history and physical is essential. A review of the patient's past medical history with focused attention on risk factors for poor wound healing or a history of scar formation is also necessary. If available, interdisciplinary collaboration with ablative surgeons and multidisciplinary tumor board review is encouraged in the setting of cancer treatment. With a team approach, the extent of extirpation can be better anticipated and guide surgical planning. Moreover, the likelihood of adjuvant treatment should be inspected and incorporated into the reconstructive treatment algorithm. Similarly, defects secondary to trauma or any history of prior reconstructive surgeries should prompt a thorough chart review as they may impact available options. A history of trauma to the forehead region or prior neurologic surgeries with pericranial flap elevation may foretell compromised supratrochlear vascular supply and warrant modification to the surgical approach. Local flaps are especially prone to the negative impact of smoking on wound healing, and as such, preoperative sessions should routinely devote time to cessation counseling. Preoperative laboratories as they pertain to wound healing and anesthetic implications should be pursued on a case-by-case basis depending on patient risk factors and institutional guidelines. Although imaging is not routinely necessary for soft-tissue defects, they are often included in cancer work-up, and thus, if available, should be reviewed for any signs of prior trauma or surgical changes.

## SURGICAL TECHNIQUE

The exact surgical technique used for the management of large nasal defects using the four-stage prelaminated forehead flap is summarized later in discussion (**Figs. 1–3**).[1] Although numerous variations exist, most described techniques share the same fundamental steps (Video 1).

### Stage 1

After induction with general anesthesia with the endotracheal tube secured to the midline lower lip, the patient is prepped and draped in standard fashion. The defect is thoroughly examined. A template of the defect is fashioned using a method of the surgeon's choosing. Various methods have been described ranging from the trimming of a pliable nonstretch material (eg, suture needle foil) to a preoperative three-dimensional printed stencil.[1] When designing the template, the surgeon must account for a slightly larger defect as the wound bed will require sharp dissection at a later stage (see **Fig. 2**D). A paramedian forehead flap is designed, incised, and elevated in the subgaleal plane based on the supratrochlear vessels. This is performed in standard fashion taking care to protect the vascular pedicle which emerges through the frontalis muscle about 2 cm above the orbital rim and carries a progressively superficial course until it is ultimately subdermal at the trichion.[19] A skin graft is harvested from the surgeon's preferred donor site. Existing publications describe the use of a split-thickness skin graft. The senior author has also used full-thickness skin grafts to lessen contraction. The size of the

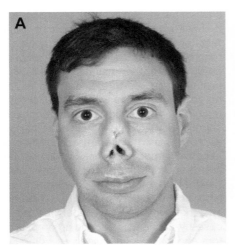 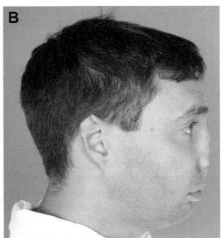

**Fig. 1.** (*A*) Preoperative studio front view of a patient who suffered from a traumatic amputation resulting in a sub-total nasal defect. (*B*) Preoperative studio profile view of a patient who suffered from a traumatic amputation resulting in a sub-total nasal defect.

graft should be oversized to account for expected contracture–particularly when a split-thickness skin graft is chosen. Most foreheads would accommodate about 5 cm graft length, as this is the average distance from the trichion to the eyebrow.[19] The harvested graft is then approximated to the galeal layer on the undersurface of the elevated forehead flap. The flap, now lined with skin graft, is inset back into its native position on the forehead in preparation for the next surgical stage. In the elapsed time, it will integrate through the classic phases of graft take: adherence, plasmatic imbibition, revascularization, and remodeling. During this time, it will undergo in-situ contracture.

## Stage 2

Although the exact optimal time is unknown, typically 4 weeks later the patient is brought back to the operating room for the second stage.[1] The previous inset is re-elevated just deep to the skin graft. The resulting elevated flap is a composite "prelaminated" paramedian forehead flap comprising an external skin paddle, subcutaneous tissue, galea/frontalis layer, and the internal skin graft layer (see **Fig. 2**B). The nasal defect edges are sharpened. Diligent attention is paid to the size and location of the nasal lining defect to ascertain the desired topography of the prelaminated layer. The template is adjusted as needed. Any excess skin graft is trimmed and areas that would otherwise overlap with intact nasal mucosa are deepithelialized. The flap is transferred to the nasal defect and further adjustments are made as necessary. As with the standard paramedian forehead flap, the pedicle width is narrowed

sufficiently to allow for tension-free rotation to reduce the risk of ischemic injury.[19] Finally, the flap is inset. The prelaminated layer is affixed to the remnant nasal mucosa, while the external forehead skin is approximated to the central midface. Given that the skin graft has already undergone contracture prior to transfer, it is expected to undergo minimal, if any, further change resulting in a stable internal reconstruction. Of note, there is no structural grafting that occurs during this stage. At this point, the reconstructed nasal components consist only of soft tissue. Thus, to prevent the early contraction of the composite PMFF, some form of temporary support must be provided. This may be with nasal packing, the use of a temporary rigid supporting structure (such as an L-shaped strut fashioned from titanium), or other means. The intention is to support the prelaminated PMFF in a fully expanded fashion during the intervening weeks prior to structural grafting.

## Stage 3

After 3 to 4 weeks, the patient is taken back to the operating room for the third stage of the reconstruction. In partial to total nasal reconstruction, this stage is arguably the most important as it ultimately dictates the structural outcome. Depending on the reconstructed subunits, incisions are made in strategic locations (eg, alar margins, sidewall, columella, and so forth) to allow for the subcutaneous elevation of the flap. The key is that the skin of the prelaminated PMFF is elevated, but the frontalis muscle along with its incorporated skin graft are left down (see **Fig. 2**C). This is possible because by this time, neovascularization has taken place to sufficiently nourish the muscle

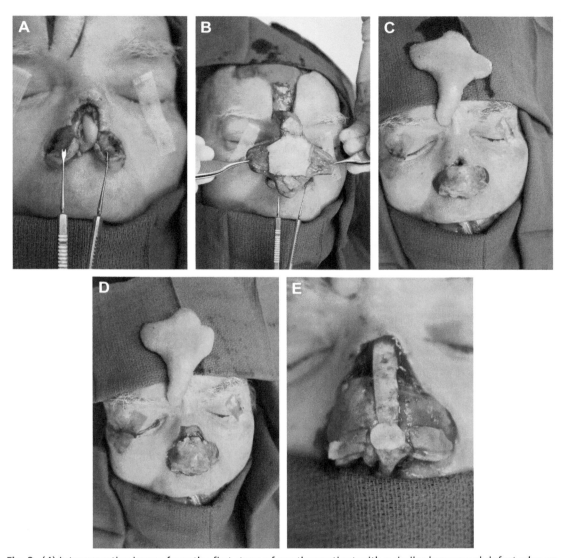

**Fig. 2.** (A) Intraoperative image from the first stage of another patient with a similar large nasal defect who underwent a prelaminated forehead flap. (B) Intraoperative image from the second stage demonstrating the appearance of the skin graft after it is re-elevated. Note there is full take, and the pliable skin has already undergone contracture and maturation. (C) Intraoperative image from the third stage demonstrating an even subcutaneous elevation to allow access to the subcutaneous fat and frontalis/galea construct. (D) Intraoperative image from the third stage demonstrating a sharp incision of the wound bed and contouring. in preparation for structural grafting. (E) Intraoperative image from the third stage where the structural framework is built using costal and auricular cartilage prior to flap redraping.

and skin graft, independent of the overlying forehead skin of the PMFF. Care is taken to ensure the elevated flap is uniform in thickness. Moreover, the flap must be thin enough to allow for appropriate contouring while not being so thin that it compromises vascular supply. With the skin paddle elevated, the surgeon has access to the subcutaneous fat and frontalis muscle/galea that are responsible for most of the flap bulk. At this time, diligent contouring can take place with the

excision of excess tissue, local tissue rearrangement, and most importantly, structural grafting for support or augmentation (see **Fig. 2**D, E). Importantly, this stage allows for the careful examination of the internal lining. Minimal further contracture, if any, should have already occurred. Areas that may be stenotic or bulky can be further thinned from the exterior and supported with structural grafting as needed. Given that the flap has already undergone neovascularization and

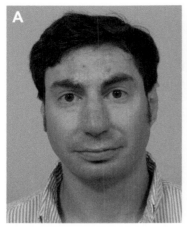
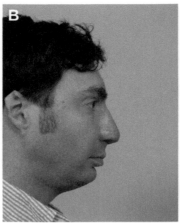
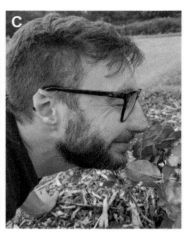

**Fig. 3.** (*A*) Postoperative studio front view of the same patient 32 months after a prelaminated forehead flap for the management of a traumatic sub-total nasal defect. Of note, the patient had a complicated course of recurrent and chronic infections causing external soft tissue loss ultimately requiring a contralateral traditional paramedian forehead flap about 13 months later. As such, there is significant forehead erythema from the patient having undergone recent dermabrasion for the second scar (image here is 19 months out from the second forehead takedown). (*B*) Postoperative studio profile view of the same patient. (*C*) Postoperative profile view of the same patient 4.5 years after initial reconstruction.

carries an independent blood supply, it can endure tissue manipulation and support implanted grafts. Once the surgeon is satisfied with the structural framework, the elevated flap can be redraped.

### Stage 4

The final stage is reserved for the division of the forehead pedicle. The exact timing is based on surgeon preference and patient factors. This may range from 2 to 4 weeks. The inset of the divided pedicle is completed in standard fashion, taking care to respect medial eyebrow alignment. The contour of the nasal root and dorsum can be adjusted as needed. Further minor adjustments of the external nose can be achieved with selective subcutaneous elevation and contouring as needed. Grafts are monitored for any migration or extrusion, particularly intranasally, as this can lead to airway obstruction or graft loss, respectively.

### Variations

Variations of the prelaminated forehead flap have been proposed. However, there is a paucity of literature on their implementation. For example, one option includes the use of a full-thickness skin graft, as opposed to a split-thickness skin graft. The former carries a reduced risk of secondary contracture and as such, would theoretically be beneficial in lining reconstruction.[1] Another variation described includes the implantation of cartilaginous grafts within the forehead concomitantly with the skin graft during the first stage.[20] This

technique, although it has the potential to omit the third stage, can be quite challenging. The exact structural framework needed is hard to predict prior to flap transfer. Moreover, with skin graft contracture in situ, there is a risk that implanted grafts migrate with the skin unpredictably, ultimately limiting reconstructive options during the second stage. The authors feel that the four-stage technique described above allows the most degree of freedom in modifying the soft tissue envelope to complement the cartilaginous construct.

### DISCUSSION

Nasal reconstruction is a challenging endeavor that requires significant attention to both form and function. The external reconstruction, in addition to its influence on the aesthetic outcome, also contributes to nasal function. For example, adequate nasal width in relation to the nasal base, sufficient nasal tip rotation, and minimal soft tissue bulk can all contribute to passage patency.[6] Although these considerations must not be underestimated, by and large, the functional outcome relies most heavily on the restoration of the internal nasal lining.

The forehead flap remains the gold standard for nasal reconstruction. The skin color and texture match render it an ideal option for the external defect.[19,21,22] Given its utility in larger defects, which by nature often also involve the nasal mucosa, modifying the technique to allow for the concomitant restoration of the lining is clearly advantageous.

The prelamination technique carries all the benefits of the paramedian forehead flap with respect to addressing the external defect, while also overcoming many of the previously summarized challenges of internal nasal lining reconstruction.

## Advantages

There are several advantages to the prelaminated paramedian forehead flap technique.

1. Unlike local techniques whereby grafts are limited in size, the use of a skin graft donor for prelamination confers unlimited availability. This is particularly important in partial to total nasal reconstruction whereby internal lining defects tend to be larger. Unlimited graft material allows the surgeon to design an oversized template that accommodates expected contracture and allows for graft excess which can be manipulated and used as needed in later stages.[6] Moreover, ample graft for internal lining ensures adequate cartilaginous graft coverage, thereby reducing the risk of extrusion.[6]
2. Importantly, the skin graft lining is thin. Therefore, the prelamination technique provides ample internal lining without introducing excessive flap bulk. Moreover, it is pliable, thereby conforming to the three-dimensional internal topography of the nasal cavity.
3. Perhaps, the most significant advantage of this technique is that it allows for the majority of secondary scar contracture to complete prior to flap transfer. In fact, this is the major premise of prelamination. Given that the skin graft contracts in situ on the forehead, the surgeon can proceed with subsequent stages of reconstruction with a lower concern for this often unpredictable variable in wound healing.[1,11] Accounting for contracture prior to flap transfer helps ensure airway patency.
4. The prelaminated paramedian forehead flap is a composite construct. As such, it allows for the transfer of an *already inset* flap that does not need bolstering. In nasal reconstruction, this is particularly useful as access is limited. With a composite flap, one can precisely arrange the internal lining.[1] Furthermore, the lining is well-vascularized prior to transfer. This allows the safe manipulation of the tissues and local rearrangement as needed at the time of inset, without compromising viability.
5. The skin graft donor site carries minimal morbidity. This is highlighted when compared with other techniques such as free vascularized tissue transfer.[6] Even endonasal flap techniques used for smaller defects often impact normal physiologic nasal function, thereby limiting their use.[9]

6. Lastly, although a minor consideration, the prelamination technique allows coverage of the forehead pedicle with a skin graft at the first stage. This mitigates slow and persistent bleeding that is often bothersome to patients and caregivers. This is particularly advantageous in the anticoagulated population who are unable to hold their medications perioperatively.

## Disadvantages

Although the prelaminated paramedian forehead flap has many distinct advantages, it does bear limitations that should be highlighted. Recall that most full-thickness nasal defects require a three-stage approach. The staged technique allows for adequate vascularity to withstand further manipulation of the structural and soft tissue framework in aesthetically sensitive areas such as the tip and alae which are the most distal.[19,22]

1. The major disadvantage to the prelaminated technique is the additional stage.[1] This stage prolongs the reconstructive process by 4 weeks, which can be bothersome to patients. As with all multiple-staged approaches, diligent consideration of patient comorbidities, age, risk factors, and the need to hold anticoagulation is necessary when deciphering the reconstructive plan.[9] Notably, patients who may require adjuvant treatment are subject to delays in starting radiation therapy or chemotherapy, which must be thoroughly discussed during counseling.
2. It is well established that the pretransfer stages of forehead flap reconstruction can be aesthetically displeasing to patients. Moreover, while the pedicle is still intact, patients are unable to wear eyeglasses.[23] In the prelaminated technique, these effects are exacerbated as pedicle takedown does not take place until the fourth and final stage, as opposed to the classic intermediate stage. Significantly, during the first stage of the prelaminated technique, the patient's primary defect remains as an open wound. In the case of large partial to total nasal reconstruction, these defects can be gruesome and disfiguring. Patients must be counseled thoroughly on this matter and assessed preoperatively for capacity to tolerate such circumstances.
3. Lastly, although split-thickness skin graft donor sites carry low morbidity, they can be aesthetically unpleasant, especially for larger defects. Harvest sites must be chosen carefully for concealment and tailored to patients' preferences. One may also consider full-thickness harvest with ex-vivo thinning, as an incision with primary closure may prove to be more inconspicuous.

## SUMMARY

A successful external nasal reconstruction relies on a stable internal milieu. Partial to the total nasal reconstruction often involves significant nasal lining loss, and its restoration can be challenging for several outlined reasons. The prelamination technique is a four-stage variation of the classic paramedian forehead flap which permits the reconstruction of the internal lining, structural framework, and external envelope concomitantly. The technique is a result of decades of lessons learned from the paramedian forehead flap. While it takes advantage of several features offered by the common forehead flap, it additionally possesses distinct features that equip it to surmount numerous challenges unique to nasal lining reconstruction. While it is a powerful technique, it does add a stage and necessitate that patients to endure the primary defect for an extended period. As such, the reconstructive surgeon must emphasize perioperative counseling, discuss alternative options, and scrutinize patient selection.

## CLINICS CARE POINTS

- Successful long-term outcomes of partial to total nasal reconstruction rely on a stable restoration of the internal nasal lining.
- The prelaminated paramedian forehead flap is an effective technique which allows concomitant internal and external nasal reconstruction.
- Pre-operative counseling focused on the advantages and disadvantages of this technique is crucial at the time of patient selection.

## DISCLOSURE

The authors have nothing to disclose.

## SUPPLEMENTARY DATA

Supplementary data to this article can be found online at https://doi.org/10.1016/j.fsc.2024.02.001.

## REFERENCES

1. Ziegler JP, Oyer SL. Prelaminated paramedian forehead flap for subtotal nasal reconstruction using three-dimensional printing. BMJ Case Rep 2021; 14(1). https://doi.org/10.1136/bcr-2020-238146.
2. Patel RG. Nasal Anatomy and Function. Facial Plast Surg 2017;33(1):3–8.
3. Rhee JS, Book DT, Burzynski M, et al. Quality of life assessment in nasal airway obstruction. Laryngoscope 2003;113(7):1118–22.
4. Taghinia AH, Pribaz JJ. Complex nasal reconstruction. Plast Reconstr Surg 2008;121(2):15e–27e.
5. Menick FJ. Nasal reconstruction. Plast Reconstr Surg 2010;125(4):138e–50e.
6. Gassner H, Sadick H, Haubner F, et al. Prelamination to reconstruct internal nasal lining. Facial Plast Surg 2013;29(5):411–6.
7. Pribaz JJ, Weiss DD, Mulliken JB, et al. Prelaminated free flap reconstruction of complex central facial defects. Plast Reconstr Surg 1999;104(2):357–65.
8. Menick FJ. The evolution of lining in nasal reconstruction. Clin Plast Surg 2009;36(3):421–41.
9. Menick FJ. Lining options in nasal reconstruction. Operat Tech Plast Reconstr Surg 1998;5(1):65–75.
10. Kim IA, Boahene KD, Byrne PJ, et al. Microvascular Flaps in Nasal Reconstruction. Facial Plast Surg. Feb 2017;33(1):74–81.
11. Pribaz JJ, Fine N, Orgill DP. Flap prefabrication in the head and neck: a 10-year experience. Plast Reconstr Surg 1999;103(3):808–20.
12. McDowell F, Valone JA, Brown JB. Bibliography and historical note on plastic surgery of the nose. Plast Reconstr Surg 1952;10(3):149–85.
13. Nelaton C. Discussion sur la rhinoplastie. Bull Mem Soc Chir 1902;28:458.
14. Gillies H. A new free graft applied to the reconstruction of the nostril. Br J Surg 1942;30(120):305–7.
15. Sinha M, Scott JR, Watson SB. Prelaminated free radial forearm flap for a total nasal reconstruction. J Plast Reconstr Aesthet Surg 2008;61(8):953–7.
16. Costa H, Cunha C, Guimarães I, et al. Prefabricated flaps for the head and neck: a preliminary report. Br J Plast Surg 1993;46(3):223–7.
17. Brackley PTH, Jones NS. The Use of a Periosteal/Forehead Flap with Sandwiched Conchal Cartilage Graft: A Novel Approach for Nasal Reconstruction in the Absence of a Nasal Septum. Plast Reconstr Surg 2002;110(3):831–5.
18. Potter JK, Ducic Y, Ellis E 3rd. Extended bilaminar forehead flap with cantilevered bone grafts for reconstruction of full-thickness nasal defects. J Oral Maxillofac Surg 2005;63(4):566–70.
19. Menick FJ. Nasal reconstruction with a forehead flap. Clin Plast Surg 2009;36(3):443–59.
20. Prasanna NS. Nasal reconstruction with pre-laminated forehead flap. Indian J Plast Surg 2017;50(3):306–9.
21. Gillies H, Millard DR. The principles and art of plastic surgery. Boston: Butterworth; 1957.
22. Menick FJ. A 10-year experience in nasal reconstruction with the three-stage forehead flap. Plast Reconstr Surg 2002;109(6):1839–55.
23. Somoano B, Kampp J, Gladstone HB. Accelerated takedown of the paramedian forehead flap at 1 week: indications, technique, and improving patient quality of life. J Am Acad Dermatol 2011;65(1):97–105.

# Total Nasal Reconstruction
## Advances in Free Tissue Transfer for Internal Lining and Structural Support

Brittany E. Howard, MD[a],*, Samip Patel, MD[b], William W. Shockley, MD[c], Joseph Madison Clark, MD[c]

### KEYWORDS

- Total nasal reconstruction • Medial femoral condyle flap • Corticoperiosteal flap • Total rhinectomy
- Innovation

### KEY POINTS

- During total nasal reconstruction, careful consideration must be given to the choice of tissue used to reestablish each nasal layer including the internal nasal lining, support structure, and external covering.
- The ideal total nasal reconstruction provides internal lining that provides a substrate for mucosalization, thereby decreasing problematic chronic crusting.
- Utilization of the medial femoral condyle flap is an innovative option for the reconstruction of the stable support structure and the nasal lining that allows for mucosalization and preserved nasal function.

## HISTORY OF NASAL RECONSTRUCTION
### Nasal Reconstruction: The First Plastic Surgery

Nasal reconstruction is considered the first elective plastic surgery.[1] It developed as a means to treat nasal amputation injuries. Several authors have provided a detailed history of nasal reconstruction.[1–4]

As the art of nasal reconstruction evolved, nasal reconstructive techniques were passed down through the generations, mostly among 3 families in India and Nepal.[3] Since these secrets were closely guarded but not recorded, it is difficult to trace the origins of the Indian method of nasal reconstruction using a midline forehead flap. However, most authors agree that this technique was practiced by the Khangiari family in Punjab in 1440 AD.[1,3]

In Italy, the Branca family devised a 6-stage operation using skin from the arm but did not record the technique. In 1502, Benedetti recorded the new procedure for nasal reconstruction, based on a pedicled flap from the arm. The Italian method was popularized by Tagliacozzi as he documented the details of the surgery along with his surgical drawings in *De Curtorum Chirurgia* in 1597.[2–4]

A description of the Indian method was published in Madras Gazette (Bombay) in 1793. The following year, a letter to the editor by "B.L." (presumed to be Colly Lyon Lucas) was published in Gentleman's Magazine (London). The author of the letter describes his observations as he witnessed the technique performed by an unnamed Indian surgeon.[1–3]

After extensive cadaveric study, Joseph Carpue became the first surgeon in Europe to perform the Indian method in 1814. Carpue's text was published in 1816 and facilitated the dissemination of this technique throughout Europe and America.[5] John Mason Warren is credited as the first American to perform the forehead flap in 1834.[1,6,7]

a Division of Facial Plastic and Reconstructive Surgery, Mayo Clinic Arizona, 5777 East Mayo Boulevard, Phoenix, AZ 85054, USA; b Division of Head and Neck Surgery, Mayo Clinic Florida, 4500 San Pablo Road South, Jacksonville, FL 32224, USA; c Division of Facial Plastic and Reconstructive Surgery, University of North Carolina, 170 Manning Drive Campus Box# 7070, Chapel Hill, NC 27599, USA
* Corresponding author.
*E-mail address:* howard.brittany@mayo.edu

Facial Plast Surg Clin N Am 32 (2024) 247–259
https://doi.org/10.1016/j.fsc.2024.01.004
1064-7406/24/© 2024 Elsevier Inc. All rights reserved.

## Development of Modern Techniques for Total Nasal Reconstruction

The nineteenth and twentieth centuries saw further innovations with a major focus on reestablishing lining. Contemporary procedures using unlined flaps were fraught with complications related to severe soft tissue contraction, resulting in marked nasal distortion. Blasius, Petrali, and Dieffenbach all proposed different methods of folding the forehead flap to provide additional skin for lining. The Gillies up-and-down flap, Converse scalping flap, and Millard seagull flap were modifications later described.[2,8] Kazanjian popularized the vertical midline forehead flap.[9]

Primary insertion of structural grafts of bone and cartilage led to exposure and extrusion of the grafts with contraction of the flap. Skin grafts were used for lining but without structural support, contraction remained a major issue. These issues directed surgeons to consider native mucosa as a solution. In 1902, de Quervain described a septal composite chondromucosal flap.[10] Other septal mucoperichondrial flaps and septal composite flaps were proposed by Kazanjian, Gilles, and Millard.[2,11,12] Gillies introduced the auricular chondrocutaneous graft, providing lining and structure for the ala and nostril.[13]

In the 1980s, Burget and Menick published 3 landmark articles that changed the course of nasal reconstruction.[14–16] They introduced many of the concepts we now take for granted (**Box 1**). These include the subunit principle, the paramedian forehead flap (formerly designed as a midline forehead flap), placing the pedicle over the supratrochlear artery, keeping the pedicle narrow (1.2–1.5 cm), multiple septal and septal composite flaps, use of the contralateral normal side as a template, and the primary insertion and fixation of multiple carefully carved cartilage grafts vascularized by mucosal lining flaps.

Burget and Menick described the marriage of beauty and blood supply: "Cartilage grafts depend on lining for vascularization; lining is dependent on a cartilage graft for support and contour."[16] One of their major tenets was the placement of cartilage grafts in nonanatomic locations: providing not only a framework for support and nasal contour but just as importantly providing resistance to soft tissue contraction. Menick developed the 3-stage folded forehead flap, which provided lining as well as cutaneous cover.[17] Because he perfected this technique, he steered away from using intranasal mucosal flaps.[18,19]

The proliferation of articles, texts, and DVDs devoted exclusively to nasal reconstruction greatly contributed to the education of reconstructive

---

**Box 1**
**Contributions to nasal reconstruction by Burget and Menick**

The subunit principle of nasal reconstruction

> The concept that discarding normal skin may enhance the final result.

> Using a template from the normal side as the subunit is reconstructed.

> Placing the forehead flap in the paramedian position.

> Aligning the pedicle with the supratrochlear artery.

> Narrowing the pedicle to 1.2–1.5 cm.

> Paramedian position and narrow pedicle allowed for greater flap length and less torque with transposition of the flap.

> Multiple intranasal mucosal flaps described (septal hinge flap, composite septal pivot flap, and so forth).

> Primary placement and fixation of carefully carved cartilage grafts (formerly cartilage grafts were placed at a secondary surgery).

> The concept that nonanatomic placement of cartilage grafts will provide contour and brace against contraction of the covering skin flap (avoiding alar retraction and weakness of the sidewall).

> Large forehead defects healed with more favorable scars when left to heal by second intention than when using skin grafts.

---

surgeons, "raising the bar" for excellence in nasal reconstruction and elevating the expertise and expectations of surgeons.[20–23]

## Advances in the Twenty-First Century

The twenty-first century has seen the continued improvement in the techniques and the results of nasal reconstruction. Formerly thought of as "too tough to tackle," reconstruction of subtotal and total nasal defects with the expectation of excellent results, has become attainable. Especially in the last 2 decades, more articles have been published on free tissue transfer (FTT) for the restoration of nasal lining.[24–29]

A recent systematic review of microsurgical techniques, as they are applied to subtotal and total nasal defects, found 11 studies suitable for review, including 232 patients.[30] The most common free flaps included auricular helical rim (n = 87), radial forearm (n = 85), anterolateral thigh (ALT; n = 30), and ulnar forearm flaps (n = 20). Other articles have proposed free fascial flaps (with secondary mucosalization), avoiding the problems with transferring skin into the nasal cavity.[31,32]

A more extensive discussion on the role of FTT as a source for lining flaps is covered later in this article.

## TOTAL NASAL RECONSTRUCTION: BASIC TENETS OF THE SURGICAL PLAN

There are few cases more challenging than total nasal reconstruction. The optimal reconstruction provides sufficient lining for airway patency and minimizes the risk of chronic nasal crusting. The structural foundation provides support and forms the shape of the nose. This framework also prevents contraction of the nasal lining tissues, "holding open" the nasal airway. A suitable skin cover is necessary for the nose to look normal with a natural skin color and texture, providing a suitable match for the surrounding skin and thin enough to reveal the contours of the aforementioned nasal subunits.

Many subtotal or total nasal defects are compound defects, involving adjacent facial units, most commonly the upper lip and cheek. When these bordering defects are full thickness or extensive in nature, it is generally best to reconstruct the lip and cheek first and delay the nasal reconstruction. Otherwise, the forces of contraction may alter the final result. Temporizing measures, such as applying skin grafts to the nasal defect, will help keep the remaining structures in place and allow the nasal defect to be addressed some weeks later. This allows the new nose to be built on a predictable and stable foundation.

As we outline a reconstructive plan for the total nasal defect, we need to consider what the "ideal total nasal reconstruction" would entail.

## IDEAL STRUCTURAL SUPPORT

As most reconstructive surgeons will agree, there is generally a variety of tissues that can provide the necessary components for the shape and foundation of the new nose. Common sources include ear composite grafts, conchal cartilage grafts, septal cartilage and bone grafts, costal cartilage grafts, and split calvarial bone grafts. Alloplastic materials are best avoided. In any given case, these resources can be used effectively to mimic the shape of the nose and provide support for a patent nasal airway.

For total nasal defects, it is useful to consider the upper half versus the lower half of the nose. Although authors differ in their preferences, a defect of the nasal bones and adjacent maxilla can be reconstructed with split calvarial bone grafts, trying to replicate the upper nasal dorsum

and sidewall. Grafts are affixed to the facial bones at the periphery of the defect. Another option for these upper nasal defects includes costal cartilage grafts or osteocartilaginous grafts.[33] These can be sutured, plated, or placed as cantilever grafts off the remaining nasal bones or frontal bone. We generally prefer an integrated L-strut with a dorsal rib graft attached to a caudal cartilaginous support such as a caudal septal replacement graft.

For the lower half of the nose, the ideal dorsum is cartilaginous, with additional support for the lower nasal sidewalls. The tip can be reconstructed by rib grafts or septal cartilage grafts. Under ideal circumstances, the alae are reconstructed with conchal cartilage grafts, sometimes accompanied by cutaneous hinge flaps for lining. Conchal cartilage grafts can be designed to provide the appropriate contour of the alar subunits and nostril margins.

In nasal reconstruction, cartilage grafts are placed in nonanatomic locations to provide not only shape and support but also serving to brace against the inevitable soft tissue contraction. These nonanatomic cartilage grafts minimize the risk of alar and sidewall collapse, alar retraction, and pin-cushion deformity.[15]

## IDEAL INTERNAL NASAL LINING

For extensive nasal defects, the biggest challenge for the surgeon is almost always how to obtain enough internal lining for the reconstruction. Lining options generally come in 3 forms: mucosa, mucosalized tissue, or epithelium (skin).

### Mucosa

The nasal mucosa consists of ciliated pseudostratified columnar epithelium conducive to mucociliary transport and effective in filtering, humidifying, and warming the inspired air. Native mucosa is the ideal lining to provide these functions and to optimize nasal airflow. In nasal reconstructive cases, the reconstitution of lining with mucosa comes from local mucosal flaps. These flaps include anteriorly based septal hinge flaps, dorsally based septal hinge flaps, septal pivot flaps, and inferior turbinate flaps.[16,34] Some authors have proposed the use of the facial artery mucosal musculature flaps for limited nasal defects.[35,36] Mucosal lining is the ideal nasal lining because it is thin and moist. Following reconstruction, it generally creates minimal to no problems with crusting, depending on the size of the septal perforation, if one has been created.

Burget and Menick had good success with septal hinge flaps and composite septal pivot flaps. The septal pivot flap was used successfully in 21 cases for subtotal and total nasal reconstruction.[16] This flap provided support for the nasal dorsum and columella, as well as providing mucosa for nasal lining.

Unfortunately, the availability of mucosal flaps is severely limited in patients with extensive nasal defects, as the donor sites have been removed with the cancer or lost with the prior trauma. In addition, they typically offer insufficient surface area for a subtotal or total nasal defect.

### Mucosalization

Mucosalization (a type of epithelialization) occurs as the native mucosa at the periphery of the defect spreads over exposed soft tissue, such as vascularized fascia, perichondrium, periosteum, or muscle from FTTs. FTTs composed of only vascularized fascia offer a flap that is thin and pliable while offering a substrate for mucosalization.[31,32,37] Pericranium has also been described for lining defects.[38] Limited defects can also be lined by dermal grafts that will also mucosalize. The lining resulting from mucosalization is considered "second best" to native mucosa. It generally allows for better nasal function, associated with less dryness or crusting and greater airway patency than a skin-lined nose.

### Epithelium

Internal nasal lining can be reconstructed with multiple sources of skin. The biggest advantage of skin for lining is the availability of large quantities. Donor sources include skin grafts, composite grafts, and local flaps. Menick has outlined several innovative methods to improve the reliability of skin grafts used for lining.[39,40] Menick also popularized the 3-stage folded forehead flap, which can bring skin lining to the lower half of the nose.[17–19] At the second stage, the lining flap is thinned, reducing the bulk that would otherwise be problematic.

Large areas of skin can also be delivered to the defect using cutaneous or compound FTTs. However, when skin is used for reconstruction of internal lining, the native ciliated columnar epithelium is replaced by keratinized squamous epithelium. Thus, the primary disadvantage of skin for internal lining is its tendency to create problems with dryness and crusting. In these patients, nasal hygiene takes on a more important role and often involves an active commitment to saline rinses and other moisturizing topical nasal agents to combat dryness.

### Bottom Line

The ideal internal nasal lining for the nose is native mucosa, generally in the form of a septal mucoperichondrial flap or composite septal pivot flap. This lining is thin, "slick" and moist, providing an optimal environment for nasal airflow while avoiding nasal dryness and crusting.

However, when total nasal reconstruction is contemplated, the use of mucosal flaps is often precluded, due to the extent of the defect and ablation of the donor sites. When available, mucosal flaps can be combined with other lining options, trying to optimize airflow and minimize dryness. Turn-in flaps (epithelial hinge flaps) also offer an excellent option for limited nasal lining. This thin lining flap is particularly useful along the alar margin, especially since this area of the nose is already lined by squamous epithelium. Flap delay is necessary when viability of epithelial hinge flaps are in question.

For many subtotal and total nasal defects, FTT offers a large surface area capable of lining even the most extensive nasal defects.

## IDEAL SKIN COVER

Following the resection of high-risk cancers, there may be situations when a split-thickness skin graft is used for a temporizing reconstruction. This allows for observation of the defect and the peripheral tissues, waiting until it is "safe" to proceed with an extensive reconstructive procedure.[41] Skin grafts provide stabilization of the remaining nasal components by minimizing the soft tissue contraction that occurs with healing by second intention. Delayed nasal reconstruction is also appropriate for extensive composite defects involving the upper lip and cheek. In these situations, it is best to reconstruct the lip, cheek, and maxilla first, providing a stable foundation for the nasal reconstruction. After stabilization of the reconstructed tissues, these mature skin grafts can also be used as epithelial hinge flaps for limited areas of nasal lining defects.

In the vast majority of cases, there is sufficient donor skin available for total nasal reconstruction. Although sometimes necessary to transfer hair with the paramedian forehead flap, there is generally enough skin for total nasal reconstruction. Even in revision cases or cases in which a second reconstruction is necessary for cancer recurrence or a new cancer, there is often sufficient skin by using a second forehead flap. In some cases, this second forehead flap may need to be delayed due to size, prior scars, pedicle placement, or an unusual vector of the flap. If 2 forehead flaps have already been used, flap delay or tissue expansion will be necessary to obtain sufficient skin to cover the newly reconstructed nose. Addressing a true deficit of forehead skin (such as burn victims) is not the focus of this article but

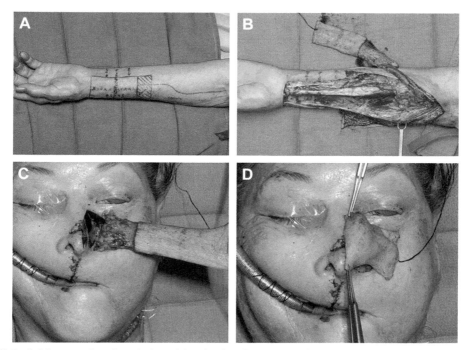

**Fig. 1.** (*A*) Radial forearm free flap designed for cheek volumizing with distal paddle planned for internal nasal lining and temporary external nasal lining. (*B*) The radial forearm free flap can be harvested with variable distal paddle with skin or as a fascial and subcutaneous fat flap based off the radial artery. (*C*) This hemirhinectomy defect was reconstructed with the radial forearm for internal lining because the free flap was already being used to restore volume and projection to the cheek that had been previously resected. The flap can use the epithelial skin paddle for lining or fascial only for lining. (*D*) Once the lining is inset, the flap can be folded back on itself for temporary external coverage to protect the vascular pedicle. Ultimately, the external nose will be reconstructed with a paramedian forehead flap.

FTT for skin cover may offer a solution. Although circumstances may dictate the use of a free flap for skin cover, the results will be suboptimal when compared with those where a forehead flap was used.

The forehead flap remains the gold standard for cutaneous cover in total nasal reconstruction. Based on imposed limitations, a delay procedure or tissue expansion may be indicated in specific cases.

## FREE TISSUE TRANSFER AS LINING FOR TOTAL NASAL RECONSTRUCTION

The use of FTT for nasal reconstruction is mostly limited to total nasal defects. For the purpose of the article, these defects comprise bilateral full thickness loss of skin, cartilage and bone, as well as mucosa. These defects often involve the upper lip and/or the cheek.[6,42] Although FTT can reconstitute each of main constituents in a

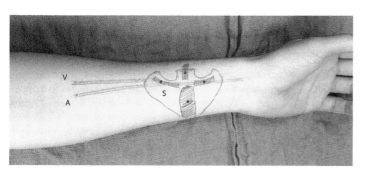

**Fig. 2.** Prelaminated flap. If harvested from the forearm, carries the same vessels as described previously. The skin paddle (S) is designed according to the defect to be repaired, in this case intranasal lining. The shaded areas (*asterisks*) represent the areas where bone and cartilage grafts will be implanted. (Facial Plastic Surgery Clinics, 19 (1), 157-162; with permission.)

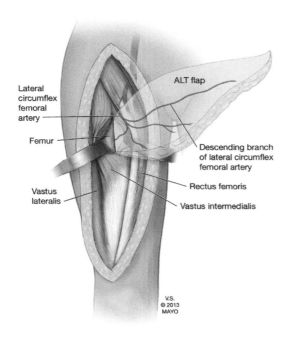

**Fig. 3.** A coronal illustration of the anterior thigh with ALT flap pedicle dissected to its origin. (From Friedrich JB, Pederson WC, Bishop AT, Galaviz P & Chang J. New Workhorse Flaps in Hand Reconstruction. Hand 7. 45-54; used with permission of Mayo Foundation for Medical Education and Research, all rights reserved.)

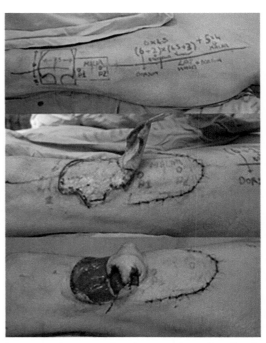

**Fig. 4.** Development of prelaminated ALT-free flap for a combined total rhinectomy and medial cheek defect. The distal portion of the skin was used for the nose and the proximal for the cheek. The skin was raised in a suprafascial plane as the nasal skin layer. The fascia was then raised separately as the inner lining layer with a costal cartilage framework interposed between the 2 layers. (*From* Bali and colleagues (2020),11 used with permission.)

single stage, ideally, each of the 3 nasal components of soft tissue envelope, osteocartilaginous framework, and mucosal lining should be considered separately. As discussed above, there are many options that may be better suited for the external skin envelope and structural framework. Here, we discuss the most challenging, often underappreciated, and likely most integral component, the FTT reconstruction of the internal nasal lining.[24] This first step in nasal reconstruction is paramount to create a patent nasal airway. In total nasal defects (due to neoplastic, traumatic, and/or prior radiation therapy), there is lack of adequate local lining options; therefore, FTT provides ample tissue for an adequate foundation in the first stage of reconstruction. Finally, the reconstructive lining must resist and prevent contracture, be thin and pliable, and support additional grafts and flaps.[43]

## TYPES OF FREE FLAPS FOR TOTAL INTERNAL LINING RECONSTRUCTION
### Radial Forearm Flap

The radial forearm flap (RFF), based off the radial artery, is the workhorse flap for total nasal reconstruction (**Fig. 1**).[24,26–31,43] Salabian and colleagues[29]

described their technique in using the infolded RFF in 47 patients in the largest series of RFF use for full thickness nasal reconstruction. Their technique shows how RFF is used as the foundation on which subsequent procedures are based. The RFF is most commonly harvested as a fasciocutaneous flap but can be harvested with bone or as a fascial flap alone. It is thin, well vascularized, with a long pedicle, and allows for design of multiple skin islands and variable skin paddle dimension.[24,26–31] It has reliable anatomy, which is resistant to atherosclerotic disease and allows for simultaneous 2-team approach. Another modification of the RFF is the multistage prelamination technique (**Fig. 2**), which allows the insertion of autologous tissues or synthetic biocompatible materials into the RFF as the first stage, creating a nasal framework buried in the arm. This construct can then be harvested at a second stage.[44,45] Drawbacks of the RFF are donor site deformity, poor graft take to the distal forearm, significant hair-bearing skin in some patients, and potential to be bulky requiring thinning.

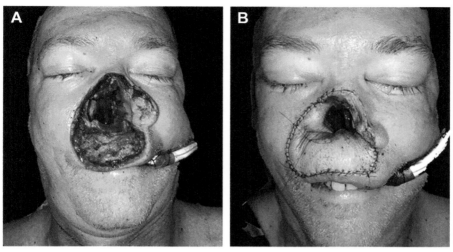

**Fig. 5.** (A) Original resection defect with oronasal fistula. (B) Radial forearm free flap used for reconstruction of the oronasal fistula, nasal floor, upper lip, and right cheek.

## Anterolateral Thigh Fascia Lata Flap

The anterolateral thigh fascia lata flap (ALTFLF), based off the lateral circumflex arterial system, is a broad, thin, and pliable flap that can provide a large source of tissue that avoids the additional bulk associated with the traditional ALT flap (**Fig. 3**).[32] Although the skin of the ALT flap can be used for internal lining, one of the benefits of this flap is the option to use its fascial layer for nasal lining instead. The fascial component, which lacks keratinized squamous epithelium, allows for remucosalization that prevents contracture and potentially avoids the need for debulking.[32] The ALTFLF can be harvested as a composite flap with skin, subcutaneous fat, and/or muscle to address adjacent defects. Overall, there is minimal associated donor site morbidity, and this flap can be considered a good alternate option to the RFF.[30,32] Additionally, similar to the RFFF, prelamination of a nasal construct within the ALT can be performed to allow a composite construct to be harvested in a second stage and transferred to the nose for reconstruction (**Fig. 4**).

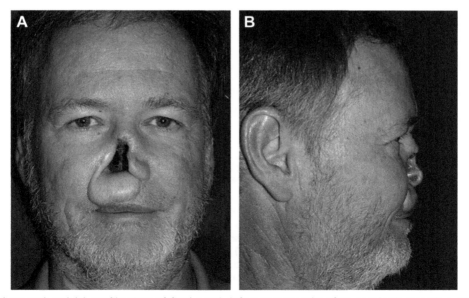

**Fig. 6.** (A) Frontal and (B) profile view of final nasal defect at 7 months after oncologic resection. Total nasal defect includes the absence of septum and turbinates with only small residual left ala and partial bony nasal vault at radix.

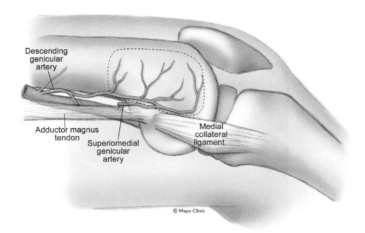

**Fig. 7.** Corticoperiosteal MFC flap based on the descending genicular artery and the superomedial genicular artery. The vascular pedicle is found immediately deep to the adductor magnus tendon. The dotted line represents the corticoperiosteal flap available for harvest, which can be up to 10–13 cm in length and 7–8 cm in width. (*From* Chieh-Ting Huang, T., Sabbagh, M. D., Lu, C. K., Steinmann, S. P., & Moran, S. L. (2019). The vascularized medial femoral condyle free flap for reconstruction of segmental recalcitrant nonunion of the clavicle. Journal of Shoulder and Elbow Surgery, 28(12), 2364-2370; with permission.)

### First Dorsal Metacarpal Flap

The first dorsal metacarpal flap is based off the dorsal metacarpal artery from the radial artery at the level of the snuffbox. It has a predictable course along the first interosseous muscle supplying skin over the first dorsal web space and the radial dorsal aspect of the index finger. Initially described for hand reconstruction, its role in nasal reconstruction is limited to subtotal nasal reconstructions due to small skin paddle size. However, it provides thin skin and has the unique ability to incorporate a double skin island design, making it very useful for intricate defects.[24,42,46] The major drawback is poor donor site cosmesis (requires skin grafting) and small vessel caliber, which may preclude microvascular anastomosis (<0.5 mm).[46]

### Ulnar Flap

The ulnar flap, based off the ulnar artery, is an alternate to the RFF because it provides similar quality tissue and can be more cosmetically appealing due to its less hirsute nature. The donor site is better concealed as well.[47,48] Drawbacks to the flap are potential risk to the ulnar nerve and the need for sacrifice of the major arterial supply to the hand, which would be contraindication in ulnar vascular dominant patients.

### Auricular Helical Flap

The auricular helical flap (AHF) is a versatile flap that can be based off the superficial temporal or postauricular arteries.[30] The ascending portion of the helix has thin skin both anterior and posterior surrounding a layer of cartilage, which can be

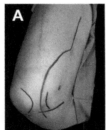 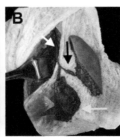 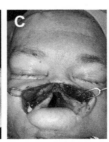 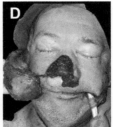 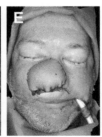

**Fig. 8.** (*A*) Right leg marked for access to MFC free flap with harvest of overlying skin paddle. (*B*) MFC corticoperiosteal flap elevated (*yellow arrow*) supplied by descending genicular vascular system (*white arrow*). Skin paddle supplied by saphenous branch (*black arrow*). (*C*) Donor site prepared with elevation of external and internal residual lining to create free edges to allow suturing and inset of the flap. (*D*) MFC flap inset at total nasal defect with periosteum sutured to residual intranasal mucosa for internal lining with interrupted chromic suture. Cortical bone osteotomized to recreate nasal pyramid and secured with miniplates across osteotomy. Bone fixed to frontal bone and bilateral maxilla with miniplates. Descending geniculate artery and vein anastomosed to right facial artery and vein. (*E*) Final flap inset with MFC flap skin paddle for initial external nasal covering.

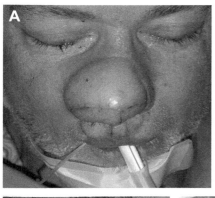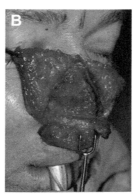

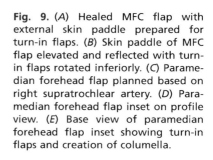

Fig. 9. (A) Healed MFC flap with external skin paddle prepared for turn-in flaps. (B) Skin paddle of MFC flap elevated and reflected with turn-in flaps rotated inferiorly. (C) Paramedian forehead flap planned based on right supratrochlear artery. (D) Paramedian forehead flap inset on profile view. (E) Base view of paramedian forehead flap inset showing turn-in flaps and creation of columella.

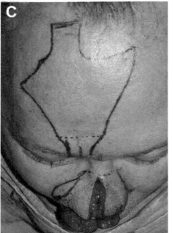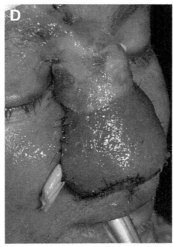

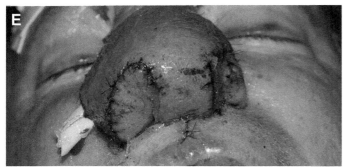

used to reconstruct the alae, and the horizontal portion of the helix can be used for alar and columellar reconstruction.[42] Advancing the AHF inferiorly to include the crus of helix can reconstruct the nostril sill.[42] Major drawback in total nasal reconstruction (TNR) is that it can only be used for unilateral or partial distal defects. Additionally, there can be significant donor site deformity of the ear.

Other free flaps to consider in nasal lining reconstruction are the temporoparietal fascia flap, dorsalis pedis flap, medial sural artery perforator flap, thoracodorsal artery perforator flap, and the medial femoral condyle (MFC) periosteal flap, which have all been reported in the literature with successful outcomes.[49,50]

## MEDIAL FEMORAL CONDYLE CORTICOPERIOSTEAL FREE FLAP

The difficulties and constraints of current techniques for TNR were highlighted for the authors' surgical team in 2016 by a patient with a locally advanced squamous cell carcinoma of the nasal cavity treated with surgical resection including

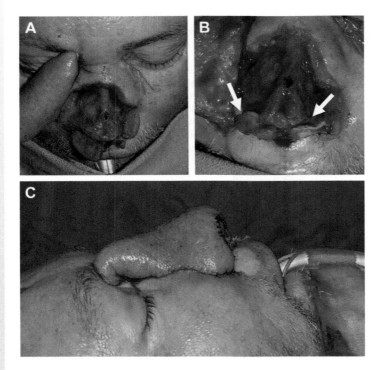

**Fig. 10.** (*A*) In third-stage surgery, the paramedian forehead flap was elevated and thinned. (*B*) Auricular cartilage grafts were placed for contouring and support along the alar rim (*white arrow*). (*C*) Paramedian forehead flap was inset with improved nasal esthetic.

upper lip, right medial cheek, hard palate, and total nasal resection (**Fig. 5**). The resultant immediate defect and oronasal fistula were reconstructed with a radial forearm free flap to create oral competency and prevent retraction (**Fig. 6**). Search for novel approaches to total nasal reconstruction identified the potential application of the MFC free flap for both nasal lining and internal nasal structure. The MFC flap is a corticoperiosteal flap from the MFC based on the descending genicular artery and the superomedial genicular artery (**Fig. 7**) with the option of a chimeric accompanying skin paddle off the saphenous branch of the arterial system.[51,52] Predominantly used as a workhorse flap for reconstruction of upper and lower extremity defects, the utilization of the MFC flap in head and neck reconstruction has been increasing given ease of harvest, low donor site morbidity, and diverse potential components (bone, periosteum, muscle, and skin). In the case of TNR, the flap has the benefit of providing thin, pliable vascularized periosteum for nasal lining that is affixed to a thin layer of cortical bone that can be rigidly fixed to stabilize and recreate the nasal pyramid.[53]

In 2012, Gaggl and colleagues[50] described utilization of the MFC concurrently with a chondrocutaneous AHF for TNR wherein the external MFC skin was used to recreate the nasal lining. Review of Gaggl and colleagues' 4 case descriptions persuaded the surgical team that this approach could potentially be applied to our patient with modifications.[50] Planned modifications from Gaggl's descriptions included reversing the flap orientation to use the periosteum for intranasal lining and use of a PMFF for skin covering. In our case, the placement of the periosteum intranasally was paramount for making the MFC flap a superior option to an RFFF because it would allow for mucosalization of the internal nasal lining.

Given the identified concerns and because this was a novel flap for the surgical team, rehearsal of the technique[54–56] was carried out in the cadaver laboratory and a conservative stepwise approach to reconstruction was planned. Ideally, the MFC flap for lining and support could be performed concurrently with a PMFF for external skin covering. However, if the MFC flap were lost, it could compromise the harvested PMFF. Thus, the decision was made to postpone the PMFF until the foundation of the nasal structure had been successfully established with the MFC flap. This created an absence of external coverage for the corticoperiosteal MFC flap. Thus, the first-stage reconstruction included harvest of MFC flap with overlying skin paddle from the right leg (**Fig. 8**). The periosteum was fixed to the residual nasal mucosa and the cortical bone was osteotomized to create a nasal pyramid. The bony pyramid was fixated using titanium miniplates (see

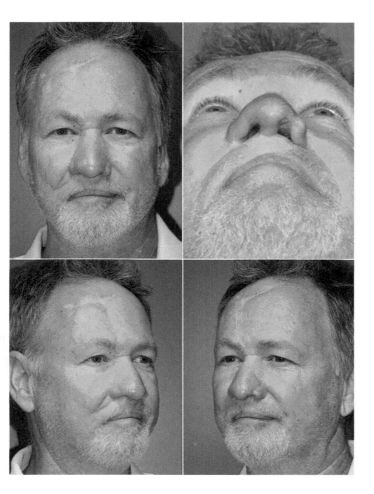

**Fig. 11.** Five-year result following total nasal reconstruction with MFC flap and paramedian forehead flap.

**Fig. 8**). The skin paddle of the MFC flap was used for external covering to allow for flap monitoring and preserve the PMFF for future use in case of flap loss. In the second-stage surgery, the external MFC skin flap was partially used for turn-in flaps to create additional lining at the nostril margins and to create the internal lining of a neocolumella. The cortical bone was modified to improve the nasal shape and a PMFF was fabricated and thinned for external nasal covering and creation of the columella (**Fig. 9**). In the third stage, the PMFF was further thinned, and auricular cartilage grafts were placed to improve nasal contours (**Fig. 10**). The PMFF was divided and inset during a fourth surgery with additional refinement of the superior flap. During that procedure, the upper lip deformity was revised using an advancement flap from the right cheek to reduce the radial forearm skin paddle. Postoperative follow-up of 5 years has shown a highly satisfactory esthetic (**Fig. 11**) and functional outcome that is notable for minimal intranasal crusting or symptoms of nasal stenosis.

During that time, the patient has undergone 3 small revision procedures to improve the nasal airway and flap refinement. Right lower extremity morbidity is minimal, as reported by the patient (playing golf regularly).

Since the completion of this case, the successful utilization of the MFC free flap with PMFF for TNR has been described by Cherubino and colleagues.[57,58] The largest case series included 8 cases with patients self-reporting both good esthetic outcomes and nasal function. All patients showed complete mucosalization of the MFC periosteal nasal lining by 6 months.[58]

## SUMMARY

We have attempted to summarize the history, the challenges and complexities, and our thoughtful consideration and development of an innovative technique for TNR. Although several options for FTT exist, we believe that the MFC flap provides an excellent option that combines a stable structure and internal lining for the upper two-thirds of the nose in TNR.

## CLINICS CARE POINTS

- Total nasal reconstruction requires creation of new internal nasal lining, internal structural support, and external skin covering.
- Skin flaps from the forehead are the gold standard for establishing the external skin covering during total nasal reconstruction.
- Internal structural support can be created with cartilage and/or bony grafting.
- Reestablishing the internal nasal lining is often the most challenging step in total nasal reconstruction; options exist including local, regional, and free flaps.
- The MFC flap is a corticoperiosteal free flap that provides an innovative option to simultaneously recreate the nasal internal support structure and a mucosal lining that allows for mucosalization during total nasal reconstruction.

## DISCLOSURE

The authors have nothing to disclose.

## REFERENCES

1. Yalamanchili H, Scafani AP, Schaefer SD, et al. The path to nasal reconstruction: from Ancient India to the present. Facial Plast Surg 2008;24:3–10.
2. Jewett BJ, Baker SR. History of nasal reconstruction. In: Baker SR, editor. *Principles of nasal reconstruction.* 2nd edition. Springer; 2011. p. 3–12.
3. Shaye DA. The history of nasal reconstruction. Curr Opin Otolaryngol Head Neck Surg 2021;29:259–64.
4. Whitaker IS, Karoo RO, Spyrou G, et al. The birth of plastic surgery: the story of nasal reconstruction from the Edwin Smith Papyrus to the twenty-first century. Plast Reconstr Surg 2007;120:327–36.
5. Carpue JC. An account of two successful operations for restring a lost nose, from the integument of the forehead. London: Longman; 1816.
6. Cannady SB, Cook TA, Wax MK. The total nasal defect and reconstruction. Facial Plast Surg Clin N Am 2009;17:189–201.
7. Warren JM. Rhinoplastic operation. Boston Med Surg J 1837;61:69–70.
8. Millard DR. Reconstructive rhinoplasty for the lower half of the nose. Plast Reconstr Surg 1974;53:133–9.
9. Kanzanjian VH. Repair of nasal defects with a median forehead flap: primary closure of the forehead wound. Surg Gynecol Obstet 1946;83:37–9.
10. De Quervain. Ueber partielle sietliche Rhinoplastik. Zentrabl Chir 1902;29:297.
11. Gillies HD, Millard DR. The principles and art of plastic surgery. Boston: Little and Brown; 1957.
12. Millard DR. Reconstructive rhinoplasty for the lower two thirds of the nose. Plast Reconstr Surg 1976;57:722–8.
13. Gillies HD. A new free graft applied to the reconstruction of the nostril. Br J Surg 1943;30:305.
14. Burget GC, Menick FJ. The subunit principle in nasal reconstruction. Plast Reconstr Surg 1985;76:239–47.
15. Burget GC, Menick FJ. Nasal reconstruction: seeking a fourth dimension. Plast Reconstr Surg 1986;78:145–57.
16. Burget GC, Menick FJ. Nasal support and lining: the marriage of beauty and blood supply. Plast Reconstr Surg 1989;84:189–203.
17. Menick FJ. A new modified method of nasal reconstruction: the Menick technique for folded lining. J Surg Oncol 2006;94:509–14.
18. Menick FJ. Nasal reconstruction with a forehead flap. Clin Plast Surg 2009;36:443–59.
19. Menick FJ. Practical details for nasal reconstruction. Plast Reconstr Surg 2013;131:613e–30e.
20. Burget GC, Menick FJ. Aesthetic reconstruction of the nose. St Louis, MO: Mosby-Year Book; 1994.
21. Baker SR. Principles of nasal reconstruction. 2nd edition. New York, NY: Springer; 2011.
22. Menick FJ. Nasal reconstruction: art and Practice. 1st edition. Philadelphia, PA: Saunders; 2009.
23. Menick FJ. Aesthetic nasal reconstruction. Principles and practice. Phoenix, AZ: Vesuvius Press Inc; 2017.
24. Walton RL, Burget GC, Beahm EK. Microsurgical reconstruction of the nasal lining. Plast Reconstr Surg 2005;115:1813–29.
25. Burget GC, Walton RL. Optimal use of microvascular free flaps, cartilage grafts, and a paramedian forehead flap for aesthetic reconstruction of the nose and adjacent facial units. Plast Reconstr Surg 2007;120:1171–207.
26. Menick FJ, Salibian A. Microvascular repair of heminasal, subtotal, and total nasal defects with a folded radial forearm flap and a full-thickness forehead flap. Plast Reconstr Surg 2011;127:637–51.
27. Menick FJ, Salibian A. Outcomes, concepts, technical refinements and challenges in the microvascular repair of full-thickness nasal defects. Plast Reconstr Surg 2023;151:1002e–14e.
28. Kim IA, Boahene KDO, Byrne PJ, et al. Microvascular flaps in nasal reconstruction. Facial Plast Surg 2017;33:74–81.
29. Salibian AH, Menick FJ, Talley J. Microvascular reconstruction of the nose with the radial forearm

flap: a 17-year experience in 47 patients. Plast Reconstr Surg 2019;144:199–210.

30. Gasteratos K, Spyropoulou G-A, Chaiyasate K, et al. Microsurgical techniques and postoperative outcomes after total nasal reconstruction. A systematic review. Ann Plast Surg 2022;88:679–86.

31. Winslow CP, Cook TA, Burke A, et al. Total nasal reconstruction. Utility of the free radial forearm fascial flap. Arch Facial Plast Surg 2003;5:159–63.

32. Seth R, Revenaugh PC, Scharpf J, et al. Free anterolateral thigh fascia lata flaps for complex nasal lining defects. JAMA Facial Plast Surg 2013;15:21–8.

33. Ciloek PJ, Hanick AL, Roskies M, et al. Osseocartilaginous rib graft L-strut for nasal framework reconstruction. Aesthetic Surg Journal 2020;40:NP133–40.

34. Baker SR, Intranasal flaps, In: Baker SR, editor. *Principles of nasal reconstruction*, 2nd edition, 2011, Springer, 211–249.

35. Heller JB, Gabbay JS, Trussler A, et al. Repair of large nasal septal perforations using facial artery myomucosal (FAMM) flap. Ann Plast Surg 2005;55:456–9.

36. Rahpeyma A, Khajehahmadi S. Facial artery musculomucosal (FAMM) flap for lining for reconstruction of large full thickness lateral nasal defects. Ann Med Surg (Lond) 2015;4:351–4.

37. Aliotta RE, Meleca J, Vidimos A, et al. Free vascularized fascia lata for total columella reconstruction. Am J Otolaryngol-Head Neck Med and Surg 2022;43:e1–4.

38. Harrison L, Seiffert M, Kadakia S, et al. Reconstruction of subtotal rhinectomy defect with chimeric paramedian-pericranial flap. Am J Otolaryngol 2019;40:445–7.

39. Menick FJ. The evolution of lining in nasal reconstruction. Clin Plast Surg 2009;36:421–41.

40. Menick FJ. The use of skin grafts for nasal lining. Clin Plast Surg 2001;28:311–21.

41. Philiips TJ. Total nasal reconstruction: a review of the past and present, with a peak into the future. Curr Opin Otolaryngol Head Neck Surg 2019;27:420–5.

42. Antunes MB, Chalian AA. Microvascular reconstruction of nasal defects. Facial Plast Surg Clin North Am 2011 Feb;19(1):157–62. PMID: 21112517.

43. Moore EJ, Strome SA, Kasperbauer JL, et al. Vascularized radial forearm free tissue transfer for lining in nasal reconstruction. Laryngoscope 2003;113(12):2078–85.

44. Pribaz JJ, Weiss DD, Mulliken JB, et al. Prelaminated free flap reconstruction of complex central facial defects. Plast Reconstr Surg 1999;104:357–65. discussion 366-367.

45. Tsiliboti D, Antonopoulos D, Spyropoulos K, et al. Total nasal reconstruction using a prelaminated free radial forearm flap and porous polyethylene implants. J Reconstr Microsurg 2008;24:449–52.

46. Beahm EK, Walton RL, Burget GC. Free first dorsal metacarpal artery flap for nasal lining. Microsurgery 2005;25:551–5.

47. Hsiao YC, Huang JJ, Zelken JA, et al. The Folded Ulnar Forearm Flap for Nasal Reconstruction. Plast Reconstr Surg 2016 Feb;137(2):630–5.

48. Kantar RS, Rifkin WJ, Cammarata MJ, et al. Free Ulnar Forearm Flap: Design, Elevation, and Utility in Microvascular Nasal Lining Reconstruction. Plast Reconstr Surg 2018 Dec;142(6):1594–9. PMID: 30489533.

49. Ramji M, Kim GY, Pozdnyakov A, et al. Microvascular lining options for subtotal and total nasal reconstruction: A scoping review. Microsurgery 2019;39:563–70.

50. Gaggl AJ, Bürger H, Chiari FM. Reconstruction of the nose with a new double flap technique: microvascular osteocutaneous femur and microvascular chondrocutaneous ear flap–first clinical results. Int J Oral Maxillofac Surg 2012 May;41(5):581–6. Epub 2012 Mar 4. PMID: 22391108.

51. Masquelet AC, Romana MC, Penteado CV, et al. Vascularized periosteal grafts: Anatomic description, experimental study, preliminary report of clinical experience. Rev Chir Orthop Reparatrice Appar Mot 1988;74(Suppl 2):240–3.

52. Sakai K, Doi K, Kawai S. Free vascularized thin corticoperiosteal graft. Plast Reconstr Surg 1991;87:290–8.

53. Rysz M, Grabczan W, Mazurek MJ, et al. Vasculature of a Medial Femoral Condyle Free Flap in Intact and Osteotomized Flaps. Plast Reconstr Surg 2017 Apr;139(4):992–7. PMID: 28350682.

54. Bürger HK, Windhofer C, Gaggl AJ, et al. Vascularized medial femoral trochlea osteocartilaginous flap reconstruction of proximal pole scaphoid nonunions. J Hand Surg Am 2013 Apr;38(4):690–700. Epub 2013 Mar 6. PMID: 23474156.

55. Doi K, Hattori Y. Vascularized bone graft from the supracondylar region of the femur. Microsurgery 2009;29(5):379–84.

56. Doi K, Oda T, Soo-Heong T, et al. Free vascularized bone graft for nonunion of the scaphoid. J Hand Surg Am 2000;25(3):507–19.

57. Cherubino M, Battaglia P, Turri-Zanoni M, et al. Medial femoral condyle free flap for nasal reconstruction: new technique for full-thickness nasal defects. Plast Reconstr Surg Glob Open 2016;4(9):e855. Erratum in: Plast Reconstr Surg Glob Open. 2016 Oct 06;4(9):e855.

58. Cherubino M, Stocco C, Tamborini F, et al. Medial femoral condyle free flap in combination with paramedian forehead flap for total/subtotal nasal reconstruction: Level of evidence: IV (therapeutic studies): Level of evidence: IV (therapeutic studies). Microsurgery 2020 Mar;40(3):343–52. Epub 2019 Nov 9. PMID: 31705579.

# Structural Support for Large to Total Nasal Reconstruction

Corin M. Kinkhabwala, MD*, Krishna G. Patel, MD, PhD

## KEYWORDS

• Structural grafting • Cartilage grafts • Nasal grafts • Nasal skeleton

## KEY POINTS

- All 3 layers of the nose (outer skin envelope, middle skeletal structure, and internal lining) must be properly reconstructed to create an esthetically pleasing and functional nose.
- It is ideal to replace framework with autologous grafts of similar size, shape, and strength.
- Nonanatomic grafting is necessary along the alar rim to prevent retraction and undesired asymmetry of the lower third of the nose.
- The final esthetic form/shape of the nose relies upon the contour of the underlying structural support.
- The timing of the placement of the structural layer is important in a multistaged total nasal reconstruction.

## INTRODUCTION: NASAL PHYSIOLOGY AND FRAMEWORK

The nose is a complex 3-dimensional structure that plays an important role in facial identity and symmetry. Its amputation (rhinokopia) and resulting disfigurement was a punishment tool used in both Eastern and Western traditions in the past, thus highlighting its importance in social identity.[1] In addition to its unique appearance, the nose facilitates olfaction and assists in humidification, warming, and filtration of inhaled air. Additionally, the nose serves as the drainage vessel of the paranasal sinuses. Therefore, reconstruction of nasal defects is important for both restoring facial esthetics as well as functionality.

When analyzing nasal defects, the nose is commonly separated into 3 layers: the outer skin envelope, the middle structural framework (osteocartilaginous support), and the inner mucosal lining. The middle framework is composed of paired nasal bones, upper lateral cartilages, lower lateral cartilages, and a cartilaginous and bony septum.

When faced with a large or total nasal defect, the reconstruction of all 3 layers is imperative. There is an intimate relationship between the 3 layers where the outer and inner layers provide vascularity, while the middle layer provides the structural support and ultimate shape.[2] The goal when reconstructing the middle layer is to design a framework that will recreate the appearance of the nose prior to insult. Failure to fully restore the middle layer may result in undesired retraction, collapse, or asymmetry after healing is complete. The goal of this article will be to outline the key components to consider when designing the middle structural framework.

## DISCUSSION
### Goals and Considerations

The goal of nasal reconstruction is to recreate as much functionality as possible while maintaining a desirable esthetic outcome. The most important function to consider is restoration of airflow. This can be challenging given the tendency for reconstructions to be bulky, and thus narrowing the

Department of Otolaryngology Head and Neck Surgery, Medical University of South Carolina
* Corresponding author. 135 Rutledge Avenue MSC 550, Charleston, SC 29425.
*E-mail address:* Kinkhabw@musc.edu

Facial Plast Surg Clin N Am 32 (2024) 261–269
https://doi.org/10.1016/j.fsc.2024.01.005
1064-7406/24/© 2024 Elsevier Inc. All rights reserved.

internal nasal passageway. Additionally, without proper structural support the nasal airway cannot be maintained. Ultimately, the final shape of the reconstructed nose will be determined by the framework of the middle structural layer recreated. When designing the middle layer, the key issues that must be addressed include

- Determining what structural components are missing and need to be replaced.
- Choosing the proper source of cartilage and or bone needed for the reconstruction.
- Deciding the appropriate timing for placing the framework/structural support.

### Sources of Framework Support

It is optimal to replace missing nasal segments with tissue that is similar in strength, size, and configuration.[3] Common sources include septal cartilage, auricular cartilage, costal cartilage or osteocartilaginous costal cartilage (autologous or cadaveric), calvarial bone, or less often, a free tissue transfer such as the osteocutaneous fibula[4] or osteocutaneous radial forearm[5] (**Table 1**). Some surgeons prefer autologous costal cartilage for younger patients when the cartilage is not yet ossified; however, multiple reports site no statistically significant difference in rates of resorption, warping, infection, or need for revision surgery.[6,7] Synthetic materials used as the source for the middle layer increase the risk of extrusion and infection.[8,9] Therefore, autologous materials should be prioritized when possible.

Grafts and vascularized flaps can either be restorative or supportive, depending on the missing tissue and the size of the defect. Restoration involves replacing nasal framework, whereas supportive refers to reinforcement of already existing cartilage or bone that may have been weakened by the injury or resection.[3] Examples of supportive grafts include nasal valve batten grafts, spreader grafts, alar rim grafts, and lateral crural strut grafts, among others.

### Auricular cartilage

Auricular cartilage can provide a versatile graft source for nasal reconstruction with minimal donor site morbidity. It can be used alone as a supportive or restorative graft, or it can be harvested as a composite chondrocutaneous graft with auricular skin (**Fig. 1**). When using a composite graft, it is important to limit the size so that "no part of the graft should be much more than 1 cm from a free edge."[10–12] Others have suggested 5 mm as the maximum distance from any part of the graft to a vascularized edge.[11] This is because composite grafts rely on a

revascularization and bridging phenomenon across the cartilage. Due to this, it is also important to limit cautery around the graft, as well as ensuring it is sufficiently immobilized to reduce the risk of shearing forces and graft failure.[13] Cartilage grafts are often harvested from the conchal bowl, which mimics the natural contour of the lower lateral cartilages. Harvesting the entire concha (concha cavum and concha cymba) can allow for restoration of the entire tip and alar subunits.[14] Contour and configuration of the concha is most similar in shape to the ala when harvested from the contralateral ear. Harvest can be performed either through an anterior or posterior auricular incision. Other auricular donor sites that can be used for nasal reconstruction include the helical crus, helical rim, antihelix, tragus, antitragus, and fossa triangularis (see **Fig. 1**). To avoid compromising the ear's appearance, 3 structures must be preserved: (1) the inferior crus of the antihelix, (2) the root of the helix, and (3) the area where the concha cavum transitions into the posterior-inferior margin of the external auditory canal.[15] Postoperatively, it is important to either secure a bolster or use full-thickness mattress sutures to minimize the risk of hematoma.

### Costal cartilage

Rib offers an abundant supply of cartilage that can provide a more rigid support compared to auricular cartilage and has the capability of being harvested either as a chondral or osteochondral composite graft. When harvested from the right, the possibility of confounding cardiac chest pain postoperatively is reduced. Harvesting from the left can be beneficial, however, when a 2-team approach is available. The graft can be taken circumferentially following perichondrial elevation or limited to just the outer lamella. Regardless of the method, care must be taken not to injure the inferior neurovascular bundle or the pleura beneath.

When using an osteochondral graft for the replacement of a dorsal septum, the bony edge is secured to the nasal bones or frontonasal suture while the cartilaginous portion extends caudally.[16] Advantages of this include lower risk of warping and the bone allows for rigid fixation using plates. Costal cartilage grafts can have early warping as soon as 15 to 60 minutes after harvest.[17] For this reason, the grafts should be carved and allowed time to warp prior to placement. Costal cartilage also has the disadvantages of ossification in older patients, a relatively distant donor site, and the risk of pneumothorax. Cartilage is most often harvested from the fifth, sixth, or seventh rib. The

**Table 1**
**Most common sources of structural support**

| Sources | Advantages | Disadvantages | Composition of the Graft |
|---|---|---|---|
| Nasal septum | • Most similar to nasal innate cartilage<br>• Thin<br>• Flexible<br>• Ease of access | • Limited supply | • Free cartilaginous graft<br>• Pedicle mucosal-cartilaginous graft |
| Auricular cartilage | • Curved shape mimics the alar subunit<br>• Easier access than costal graft<br>• Can provide range of support grafts<br>• Low donor site morbidity | • Limited supply<br>• Less resilient than other cartilage sources | • Cartilaginous graft<br>• Skin-cartilage composite graft |
| Costal cartilage | • Robust supply<br>• Strong<br>• Flexible (if young)<br>• Able to control thickness of graft | • Warp potential<br>• Increased donor site morbidity (pain, pneumothorax, hematoma)<br>• Potential ossification centers within graft with age | • Osseocartilaginous composite graft<br>• Cartilaginous graft |
| Cadaveric costal cartilage | • Robust supply<br>• Ease of availability (depending on center)<br>• No harvest site morbidity | • Brittle<br>• Less strong compared to autologous<br>• Higher resorption in high tension areas | • Cartilaginous graft |
| Split calvarial bone graft or iliac crest graft | • Robust supply<br>• Strong<br>• Membranous bone (calvarium) lowest risk of resorption | • Non-flexible<br>• Requires stabilization with plates or drill holes for suturing<br>• Increased donor site morbidity | • Osseous graft |
| Free tissue transfer | • Vascularized flap<br>• Strong<br>• Robust supply<br>• Can be multilayered (+lining or cover) | • Bulky<br>• Increased donor site morbidity<br>• Possible flap failure<br>• Difficult to refine shape | • Osseo-cutaneous composite graft |

central portion of these ribs is preferred by some surgeons, as it is more straight and less prone to warping.[18] The eleventh and twelfth free-floating ribs are also an option due to their straighter orientation and lower risk of warping.[19]

### Septal cartilage
While costal and auricular cartilages provide readily available and robust sources of graft material, septal cartilage remains an optimal graft source given its similarity in flexibility and thinness to the lower and upper lateral cartilages. Using septal cartilage also reduces the morbidity of

separate graft harvest sites. It is useful for restoring framework of the nasal dorsum, tip, columella, and caudal aspect of the nasal side walls.[14] Septal cartilage grafts have less of a propensity to warp compared to costal cartilage and provide more rigidity compared to auricular sources. If needing natural curvature similar to that of an auricular graft, it can be scored or fixated to provide some additional contouring. It is harvested through a standard septoplasty incision, unless a large defect is already present. Its primary limitation in large defect nasal reconstruction is lack of availability.

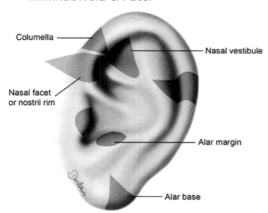

**Fig. 1.** Common donor sites for composite grafts used in nasal reconstruction. The unlabeled sites of the tragus and helical rim are good choices for alar rim or columellar defects. (Jewett, B.S., Baker, S.R. (2011). Skin and Composite Grafts. In: Principles of Nasal Reconstruction. Springer, New York, NY. https://doi.org/10.1007/978-0-387-89028-9_9.)

### Bone grafts

When there is a partial or total bony pyramid defect, a bone graft is often required. Options include iliac crest, osteochondral rib, and calvarium. Today, the most commonly used is the split-calvarial graft, which is harvested from the outer table of the parietal bone[20] (**Fig. 2**). It can be harvested relatively easily with a well-hidden scar and often is associated with less postoperative pain compared to the iliac crest and rib. Lastly, membranous bone (calvarium) has been shown to have reduced resorption and have greater survivability compared to endochondral bone (rib, iliac crest).[21–26] During harvest, it is important to avoid injury to the superior sagittal dural sinus, which runs beneath the sagittal suture and can be as wide as 1.5 cm. As such, harvest should be at least 2 cm from the midline.[27–30]

Grafts can be fixed to the frontal bone with fixation plates or to the remaining nasal bones. It is important when using a bone graft to cover all sides with soft tissue to reduce the risk of infection. Because of this, both lining flaps and external skin flaps are recommended.

In cases of large oncologic resections with prior radiation history, comorbid or immunocompromised patients with higher risk for infection, or large defects involving the maxilla, a free tissue transfer or vascularized graft may be preferred. Vascularized tissue will be more resistant to infection, necrosis, and resorption. A free flap can also provide additional cover or lining for the reconstruction. The osteocutaneous radial forearm flap is one such example that offers a thin bone stock for nasal framework restoration while providing tissue to replace the lining or cover. The bone can be osteotomized to create a new L-strut, and by using an additional skin graft to replace either the cover or lining, it has the potential to be a 1-stage surgery for large nasal defects.[5]

### Analysis of the Anatomic Defect/Designing the Framework

The nasal defect can be characterized using the subunit principle previously described by Burget and Menick,[31] where the external nasal anatomy is subdivided into the paired lateral sidewalls, paired alar lobules, paired soft tissue triangles, nasal dorsum, nasal tip, and columella. These divisions are based on contours created by highlights and shadows. Once the borders of the defect are noted, the missing tissue is characterized. With large nasal reconstruction planning, a template of the missing subunits is typically designed. The underlying framework and grafts often mimic the shape of the designed template.

**A**

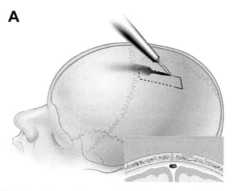

**B**

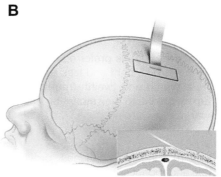

**Fig. 2.** Split-calvarial graft harvest. (*A*) A side-cutting bur is used to drill a trough at the periphery of the bone graft. (*B*) The medial trough is beveled with a cutting bur to allow the placement of an oscillating 90° saw blade, which traverses diploic space under the graft. A chisel is used to release the bone graft. (Jewett, B.S., Baker, S.R. (2011). Skin and Composite Grafts. In: Principles of Nasal Reconstruction. Springer, New York, NY. https://doi.org/10.1007/978-0-387-89028-9_9.)

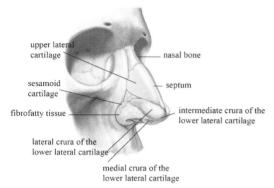

upper lateral cartilage

nasal bone

sesamoid cartilage

septum

fibrofatty tissue

intermediate crura of the lower lateral cartilage

lateral crura of the lower lateral cartilage

medial crura of the lower lateral cartilage

**Fig. 3.** Nasal cartilages. (Naficy, S., Baker, S.R. (2011). Bone Grafts. In: Principles of Nasal Reconstruction. Springer, New York, NY. https://doi.org/10.1007/978-0-387-89028-9_8.)

In normal nasal anatomy, all nasal subunits contain a rigid framework with the exception of the soft tissue triangle and the ala (**Fig. 3**). The nasal bones support the undersurface of the upper half of the dorsum and lateral sidewall subunits. The septum, upper lateral cartilages, and lower lateral crura support the lower half of the dorsum and the lateral sidewall subunits. The intermediate crura and the medial crura of the lower lateral cartilages support the nasal tip subunit and columella, respectively. When reconstructing a nasal defect, all subunits must have a rigid underlying framework. Therefore, nonanatomic grafts must be placed within the alar and soft tissue triangles. In all other areas of the nose, the framework should be replaced and take the shape of the subunit it supports[31] (**Fig. 4**).

For large midline defects, costal cartilage is generally preferred to provide a robust enough graft. It can be secured cephalad to the remaining nasal bones in a tongue-and-groove-style joint or as a cantilevered onlay graft. This dorsal segment can either be purely cartilaginous or osseocartilaginous if missing nasal bones require reconstruction. If there are remaining nasal bones, a subperiosteal pocket is created and the nasal bones are rasped down to accommodate the graft and promote integration.[32] An L-strut can then be created by extending the graft caudally to a separate columellar strut, which is sutured to the spine or maxillary crest. These can be fixed together as a tongue-and-groove joint. Some investigators describe a maximum width of 4 mm for the caudal segment to reduce the risk of warping.[32] Another option available when the nasal bones are preserved is using 2 extender spreader grafts to replace the dorsal septum. Holes are drilled into the caudal aspect of the nasal bones and then secured to the grafts with a 4-0 polydioxanone suture. These are then secured to a caudal septal replacement graft, which is sutured to the spine.[33] After replacing the septum, additional lateral grafts can be secured to the dorsal graft to replace the sidewalls and/or lower lateral cartilages (**Fig. 5**). If the dorsum is reconstructed with an onlay graft, the edges should be tapered to prevent unnatural angles at the junction of the lateral sidewall and dorsal subunits.

In total nasal defects, bone grafts (often split-calvarial) and vascularized bone are preferred for recreating the dorsal support. Split-calvarial non-vascularized bone grafts have a relatively low complication rate and can provide a lasting rigid augmentation for nasal reconstruction[34–36] (**Fig. 6**). The bone requires fixation to the surrounding bone using either titanium plate-screw systems or bioresorbable screws. During restoration of the entire bony pyramid, the calvarial bone graft can either be split into 3 parallel segments (dorsum plus 2 mirror-image grafts for the sidewalls) or 2 parallel segments without a separate dorsal piece

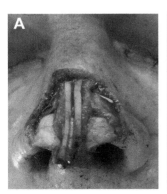
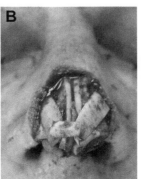
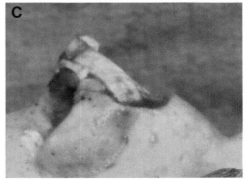

**Fig. 4.** (*A*) Frontal view. Septal cartilage is used for bilateral extended spreaders and septal extension graft. Auricular cartilage is used to create nonanatomic rim grafts; (*B*) Frontal view. Autologous costal cartilage is used to re-establish sidewalls in addition to a tip graft; (*C*) Profile view following replaced framework. Note the tip graft placed to enhance nasal tip projection.

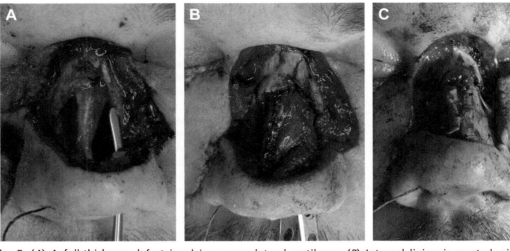

**Fig. 5.** (*A*) A full-thickness defect involving upper lateral cartilages. (*B*) Internal lining is created with local mucosal flaps. (*C*) The middle framework is replaced with autologous costal cartilage carved in the form of the lateral sidewall subunits.

or fixation plate. Osteochondral costal grafts are also an appropriate option. In this technique, bony and cartilaginous ribs can be fashioned together to create 1 composite costal dorsal strut that can be secured to the frontal bone, and a third piece of costal cartilage can create a columellar strut caudally. When there are minimal nasal bone remnants remaining, it is often easier to drill the remaining nasal bones away and create a small trough in the nasal process of the frontal bone as a recipient site for whatever graft is chosen.[30]

When lateral sidewall subunits are involved, broader rectangular shaped grafts are designed.

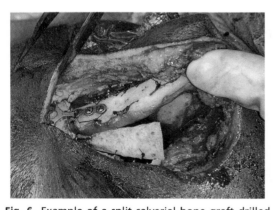

**Fig. 6.** Example of a split-calvarial bone graft drilled to simulate the shapes of the dorsal and sidewall subunits. Drill holes were placed for suture stabilization. The dorsal graft was stabilized to frontal process with titanium plate fixation. Internal lining was then placed using free tissue transfer and supported onto the framework.

The lateral edge of the graft is secured along the lateral aspect of the pyriform aperture. This prevents medialization or collapse into the nasal passageway. The caudal aspect of the graft should be positioned posterior (deep) to the cephalic edge of the lower lateral (alar) cartilage to preserve the natural relationship and contour of the supra-alar groove. If lining is needed in addition to support, septal cartilage can be harvested as a composite septal mucoperichondrial hinge flap to provide lining and support for the nasal sidewall and roof of the middle vault.[37] To improve positioning of the cartilage into the sidewall, however, the cartilage is often separated from the underlying hinge flap. When there is not enough septal cartilage for the sidewall or there is also nasal bone missing, a brace can be created from the ethmoid perpendicular plate with attached cartilage. This both supports the middle vault and provides a platform for glasses.[37] Late complications of lateral nasal side wall fistulas are often due to inadequate structural middle layer support.

If the alar subunit is missing, a nonanatomic alar replacement graft (auricular cartilage, most often) can be used. As previously stated, the nonanatomic alar replacement graft should be positioned with the caudal edge along the alar rim and the cephalic edge superficial to the upper lateral cartilage graft.[3] The alar graft is oriented at roughly 90° to the sagittal plane in a nonanatomic fashion, in contrast to the anatomic 45° angles of innate lateral crural anatomy. Auricular and septal cartilages are most often the source for alar replacement grafts given their ideal properties of flexibility, thinness, and contour. The purpose of

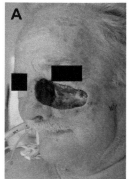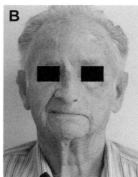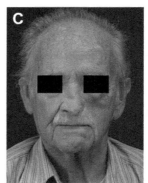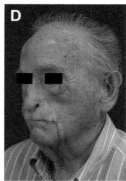

**Fig. 7.** Example of alar retraction following radiation in a patient who received lateral wall reconstruction without alar rim grafting. (*A*) Nasal sidewall defect. (*B*) Following sidewall reconstruction and paramedian forehead flap for cover. (*C and D*) Following radiation with resulting alar retraction.

these nonanatomic grafts is to prevent future collapse or retraction of the alar rim, particularly in patients who require radiation (**Fig. 7**).

For nasal tip reconstruction, the profile height of the tip graft ideally projects further than the height of the dorsal graft. This anatomic relationship of the grafts mimics the normal anatomic relationship between the cartilaginous domes and the cartilaginous dorsum. Increased projection at the nasal tip can be achieved using a Peck-style graft on top of the new domes[38] (see **Fig. 4**).

### Timing Placement of Structural Grafts

Often, large defects involve the use of paramedian forehead flaps. This means there are likely multiple stages involved in the reconstruction and, therefore, multiple available timepoints to introduce structural support. When possible, earlier placement of structural support is best to prevent natural wound contraction. Therefore, if the internal and external layers have independent blood supply, it is often safe to place the middle structural support layer at the first surgical stage of the reconstruction. However, if a full-thickness skin graft or folded forehead flap is employed, the structural layer should be delayed to the second stage of the reconstruction. This second stage is often when the outer layer forehead flap is contoured and debulked. This is the most ideal time to ensure that all structural grafts are in place and the structural framework creates the desired shape of the nose. This also affords the opportunity to reposition any grafts placed at the primary stage into a better position.

### SUMMARY

Reconstruction of the nasal osteocartilaginous framework involves both the replacement of missing tissue and the support of remaining subunits. Grafts should be similar strength, size, and shape as the missing tissue and autologous when possible. Auricular grafts can be either cartilaginous or composite and are most often utilized to reconstruct the nasal tip and ala. Nonanatomic grafts along the alar rim aid in preventing future retraction or collapse of the nasal airway. Costal chondral grafts provide robust midline septal support and can also be harvested as osteochondral grafts when additional bone is required. The preferred donor site for large bony defects is the split-calvarial, which is particularly resistant to resorption. Structural grafts should be placed as early as possible and require a vascularized lining to support survival.

### CLINICS CARE POINTS

- The purpose of the structural layer is to
  - Ultimately drive the final shape of the nose
  - Optimize function by providing structural support of the nasal airway
  - Prevent retraction or collapse
  - Prevent fistula formation from inadequate nasal wall support
- Keys to proper reconstruction of the middle layer are
  - Assess the defect and determine what structural support is missing
  - Provide structural support to all subunits of the nose
  - Design and create the structural support to mimic the shape of the missing subunit
  - Choose the optimal source for cartilage or bone grafts

- ○ Place structural support as early as possible as long as there is a vascularized outer and inner layer to cover the grafts

## DISCLOSURE

No authors have financial or relevant conflicts of interest to disclose.

## REFERENCES

1. Mazzola IC, Mazzola RF. History of reconstructive rhinoplasty. Facial Plast Surg 2014;30(3):227–36.
2. Menick FJ. Aesthetic nasal reconstruction: principles and practice. Frederick J. Menick, M.D.; 2017.
3. Naficy S. and Baker S.R., Structural support, Principles of Nasal Reconstruction, 2011. 47-64, chapter 5.
4. Nakayama B, Takeuchi H, Takeuchi E, et al. Subtotal nasal reconstruction for ethmoid sinus cancer defect using a fibula osteocutaneous free flap. J Reconstr Microsurg 2006;22(06):451–6.
5. Koshima I, Tsutsui T, Nanba Y, et al. Free radial forearm osteocutaneous perforator flap for reconstruction of total nasal defects. J Reconstr Microsurg 2002;18(7):585–8. ; discussion 589-590.
6. Saadi R, Loloi J, Schaefer E, et al. Outcomes of cadaveric allograft versus autologous cartilage graft in functional septorhinoplasty. Otolaryngology-Head Neck Surg (Tokyo) 2019;161(5):779–86.
7. Vila PM, Jeanpierre LM, Rizzi CJ, et al. Comparison of autologous vs homologous costal cartilage grafts in dorsal augmentation rhinoplasty: a systematic review and meta-analysis. JAMA Otolaryngology–Head & Neck Surgery 2020;146(4):347–54.
8. Loyo M, Ishii L. Safety of alloplastic materials in rhinoplasty. JAMA Facial Plastic Surgery 2013;15(3):162–3.
9. Keyhan SO, Ramezanzade S, Yazdi RG, et al. Prevalence of complications associated with polymer-based alloplastic materials in nasal dorsal augmentation: a systematic review and meta-analysis. Maxillofac Plast Reconstr Surg 2022;44(1):17.
10. Ruch M. Utilization of composite free grafts. J Int Coll Surg 1958;30(2):274–5.
11. Ballantyne D, Converse J. Vascularization of composite auricular grafts transplanted to the chorioallantois of the chick embryo. Transplant Bull 1958;22:373–6.
12. Becker O. Extended applications of free composite grafts. Transactions-American Academy of Ophthalmology and Otolaryngology American Academy of Ophthalmology and Otolaryngology 1960;64:649–59.
13. Gjorup CA, Moeller MP, Asklund C, et al. Versatility of composite grafts for nasal defects - a case series. Case Reports Plast Surg Hand Surg 2022;9(1):236–48.
14. Naficy S. and Baker S.R., Cartilage grafts, Principles of Nasal Reconstruction, 2011. 103-120. Chapter 7.
15. Lee M, Callahan S, Cochran CS. Auricular cartilage: harvest technique and versatility in rhinoplasty. Am J Otolaryngol 2011;32(6):547–52.
16. Chait LA, Becker H, Cort A. The versatile costal osteochondral graft in nasal reconstruction. Br J Plast Surg 1980;33(2):179–84.
17. Moretti A, Sciuto S. Rib grafts in septorhinoplasty. Acta Otorhinolaryngol Ital 2013;33(3):190–5.
18. Lee M, Inman J, Ducic Y. Central segment harvest of costal cartilage in rhinoplasty. Laryngoscope 2011;121(10):2155–8.
19. Ansari K, Asaria J, Hilger P, et al. Grafts and implants in rhinoplasty—techniques and long-term results. Operat Tech Otolaryngol Head Neck Surg 2008;19(1):42–58.
20. Jackson IT, Smith J, Mixter RC. Nasal bone grafting using split skull grafts. Ann Plast Surg 1983;11(6):533–40.
21. Zins JE, Whitaker LA. Membranous versus endochondral bone: implications for craniofacial reconstruction. Plast Reconstr Surg 1983;72(6):778–85.
22. Kusiak JF, Zins JE, Whitaker LA. The early revascularization of membranous bone. Plast Reconstr Surg 1985;76(4):510–6.
23. Smith JD, Abramson M. Membranous vs endochondrial bone autografts. Arch Otolaryngol 1974;99(3):203–5.
24. Motoki DS, Mulliken JB. The healing of bone and cartilage. Clin Plast Surg 1990;17(3):527–44.
25. Lin KY, Bartlett SP, Yaremchuk MJ, et al. The effect of rigid fixation on the survival of onlay bone grafts: an experimental study. Plast Reconstr Surg 1990;86(3):449–56.
26. LaTrenta GS, McCarthy JG, Breitbart AS, et al. The role of rigid skeletal fixation in bone-graft augmentation of the craniofacial skeleton. Plast Reconstr Surg 1989;84(4):578–88.
27. Frodel JL Jr, Marentette LJ, Quatela VC, et al. Calvarial bone graft harvest. Techniques, considerations, and morbidity. Arch Otolaryngol Head Neck Surg 1993;119(1):17–23.
28. Sullivan WG, Smith AA. The split calvarial graft donor site in the elderly: a study in cadavers. Plast Reconstr Surg 1989;84(1):29–31.
29. de Souza Fernandes AC, Neto AIT, de Freitas AC, et al. Dimensional analysis of the parietal bone in areas of surgical interest and relationship between parietal thickness and cephalic index. J Oral Maxillofac Surg 2011;69(11):2930–5.
30. Naficy S. and Baker S.R., Bone grafts, Principles of Nasal Reconstruction, 2011. 121-132. Chapter 8.
31. Burget GC, Menick FJ. The subunit principle in nasal reconstruction. Plast Reconstr Surg 1985;76(2):239–47.
32. Ciolek PJ, Hanick AL, Roskies M, et al. Osseocartilaginous rib graft L-strut for nasal framework reconstruction. Aesthetic Surg J 2019;40(4):NP133–40.

33. Toriumi DM. Subtotal septal reconstruction: an update. Facial Plast Surg 2013;29(06):492–501.
34. Powell NB, Riley RW. Cranial bone grafting in facial aesthetic and reconstructive contouring. Arch Otolaryngol Head Neck Surg 1987;113(7):713–9.
35. Powell NB, Riley RW. Facial contouring with outer-table calvarial bone: a 4-year experience. Arch Otolaryngol Head Neck Surg 1989;115(12):1454–8.
36. Smolka W, Eggensperger N, Kollar A, et al. Midfacial reconstruction using calvarial split bone grafts. Arch Otolaryngol Head Neck Surg 2005;131(2):131–6.
37. Burget GC, Menick FJ. Nasal support and lining: the marriage of beauty and blood supply. Plast Reconstr Surg 1989;84(2):189–202.
38. Peck GC. The onlay graft for nasal tip projection. Plast Reconstr Surg 1983;71(1):27–39.

# Nuances in Forehead Flap Reconstruction for Large Nasal Defects

Betsy Szeto, MD, MPH, Hannah Jacobs-El, MPH, Stephen S. Park, MD*

## KEYWORDS

• Nasal reconstruction • Forehead flap • Nasal defects

## KEY POINTS

- The forehead flap is a workhorse resurfacing flap used for the reconstruction of large nasal defects.
- The forehead flap has an excellent color and texture match, acceptable donor site morbidity, and robust and independent blood supply that can support both structural and internal lining grafts.
- Defect preparation should consider the nasal esthetic subunits.
- Various nuances of this technique are discussed in this article and are the guiding principles for forehead flap reconstruction of large nasal defects.

## BACKGROUND/INTRODUCTION

Successful nasal reconstruction combines a mastery of esthetics and surgical techniques to create a functionally stable nose that is visually inconspicuous. The forehead flap is a time-tested resurfacing flap with an excellent color and texture match, acceptable donor site morbidity, and robust and independent blood supply that can support both structural and internal lining grafts. It is a common dogma among algorithms for nasal reconstruction that the forehead flap should be chosen for defects greater than 1.5 cm; however, smaller defects on smaller noses, for example, Asian patients, will occasionally require this flap for optimal resurfacing. It is versatile and can itself be used for restoration of internal lining by folding the distal aspect.[1] A double forehead flap has also been described for reconstruction of larger composite nasal defects.[2]

This article will highlight specific nuances of the forehead flap, some of which may dispel prior myths and even aphorisms. Similar to many things in medicine, certain beliefs and practices can be passed down as dogma, only to be challenged and possibly disproven many years later.

## DEFECT PREPARATION AND TEMPLATE CREATION

During defect analysis and preparation, it is very useful to draw the nasal esthetic subunits[3] directly onto the nose, taking care to preserve straight lines and sharp corners at the junction of the subunits. The defect is usually manipulated to some degree with the specific goal of controlling the final resultant scars and making them as inconspicuous as possible. It does not always result in the complete excision of esthetic units but the mental exercise can prove to be very beneficial. The defect is not always enlarged to complete a subunit; at times, a small local flap can be designed to partially close the defect and alter the shape in a favorable way. For example, for a defect that encompasses the nasofacial junction, a cheek advancement flap should be brought up to the nasofacial junction to reduce the size of the defect (**Fig. 1**). Once again, the edges of the defect should be squared off to ensure straight lines and crisp corners at subunit junctions (**Fig. 2**). Finally, the depth of the defect is usually taken down to the perichondrium and periosteum of the nose. The local flaps are also elevated and

Department of Otolaryngology – Head and Neck Surgery, University of Virginia, PO Box 800713, Charlottesville, VA 22908, USA
* Corresponding author.
*E-mail address:* SSP8A@uvahealth.org

Facial Plast Surg Clin N Am 32 (2024) 271–279
https://doi.org/10.1016/j.fsc.2023.11.002

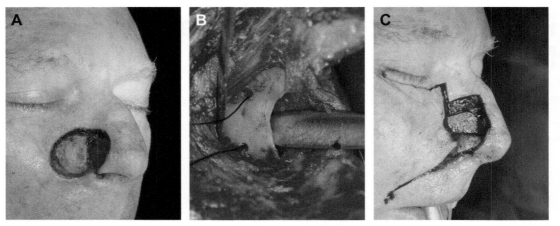

**Fig. 1.** (*A*) Defect of right nasal sidewall and ala, extending onto right cheek, encompassing nasofacial junction. (*B*) Holes were drilled into the frontal process of the maxilla to secure a planned cheek advancement flap. (*C*) The cheek advancement flap is brought up to the nasofacial junction to reduce the size of the defect.

transposed in that plane of dissection, which allows skin movement with minimal cartilage distortion. A deeper nasal defect allows for a thicker forehead flap, which can include portions of the forehead galea and frontalis muscle. This is also when various cartilage sutures can be placed with wide exposure. For example, nasal airflow can be enhanced by placement of *flaring sutures* across the upper lateral cartilages.[4] After defect preparation, a template is made of the final

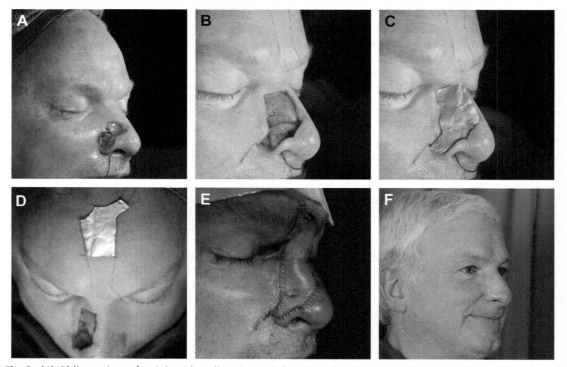

**Fig. 2.** (*A*) Oblique view of a right sidewall and alar defect. (*B*) After defect modification with consideration of esthetic subunits principle. Edges of the defect are squared off to ensure straight lines and crisp corners. (*C*) Template made from aluminum package from a suture. (*D*) The template is placed in the midline of the forehead and traced onto the forehead. (*E*) Immediate postoperative photo with forehead flap in situ. (*F*) Four months after reconstruction.

cutaneous defect. The aluminum package from a suture is used to create a 3-dimensional template of the defect (see **Fig. 2**C). The template is then transferred to the forehead where it is flattened and traced out. The vertical position is determined by measuring the distance from the medial aspect of the brow down to the nasal defect. One should err on the side of having excess pedicle length to ensure that the flap can reach the defect without tension.

## FLAP DESIGN: MIDLINE VERSUS PARAMEDIAN

It is widely accepted that the blood supply to the forehead flap is primarily through the supratrochlear artery.[5] It is now accepted that the primary driver of this flap is more than that single artery but also based on a rich perfusion pressure from the collateral flow off the angular artery and dorsal nasal arteries.[5–7]

It was originally thought that the flap pedicle needed to be wide enough to capture both right and left supratrochlear vessels for adequate perfusion of the flap. The pedicle of this *median* forehead flap was designed as such[8] (**Fig. 3**A). It was later noted that a single supratrochlear vessel was sufficient to perfuse the flap,[9–12] and that, on the contrary, a wider pedicle would result in kinking of the pedicle, impeding perfusion. Furthermore, a narrower pedicle would allow for an improved arc of rotation. This *paramedian* design created a straight pedicle that ascends vertically from the supratrochlear notch or foramen[13] (**Fig. 3**B). The skin paddle would be harvested from this paramedian position, resulting in a donor site scar that is vertically linear and paramedian. This is the most common design. The donor site generally heals well. The skin paddle

is off-center and that can be beneficial in patients with a prominent widow's peak. Hair on the distal skin paddle is often a nuisance and may require additional steps to treat, such as depilation during flap elevation or use of future laser treatments.[1,14] Additionally, the linear pedicle would offer an improved vascular design, especially important in individuals with small vessel disease, for example, smokers. Alternatively, the skin paddle can be designed in the exact midline of the forehead, whereas the pedicle then narrows as it proceeds inferiorly and finally diverts to one side inferiorly. This *midline* design is a hybrid that is still a unilateral forehead flap, based on the take-off of a single supratrochlear pedicle[15] (**Fig. 3**C). The pedicle is not vertically linear but rather has an arc to the design along the glabellar area. In theory, this arc would be less optimal in terms of capturing all collateral vessels but the reliability of this flap has been shown to be consistent. Additionally, the curved arc to the pedicle gives some additional length to the flap that can prove to be very useful when there is a low hairline and the flap must reach to the caudal border of the nose. The resultant scar will be in the midline of the forehead and is more favorable and inconspicuous for 2 reasons. First, it bisects the face and is more consistent with facial esthetic subunits because the face is visually divided into 2 halves. Second, although the scar is perpendicular to the horizontal forehead furrows, the midline forehead flap leaves a midline vertical donor site scar and tends not to disrupt these because there is a natural divergence of the frontalis muscle and its corresponding horizontal furrows across the forehead.

As previously discussed, a narrow pedicle allows for an improved arc of rotation and avoids buckling of the blood supply to the flap. It has

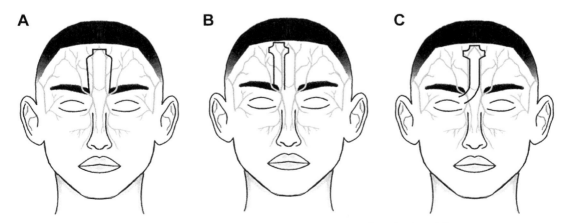

**Fig. 3.** (*A*) Median forehead flap. (*B*) Paramedian forehead flap. (*C*) Midline forehead flap.

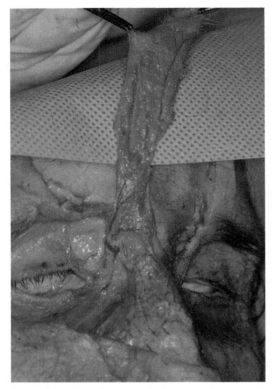

**Fig. 4.** This cadaveric anatomic dissection illustrates the rich collateral circulation along the glabellar and medial brow areas. The supratrochlear artery, a branch of the internal carotid artery, was not injected. The right-sided facial artery, a branch of the external carotid, was cannulated and injected, demonstrating a robust arcade of vessels within the midline forehead flap.

previously been shown that the pedicle can be safely narrowed to 1.2 to 1.5 cm without compromising flap viability.[16,17]

Generally, a pedicle contralateral to the nasal defect is recommended because it requires a smaller arc of rotation, resulting in less kinking of the pedicle and improved perfusion to and venous return from the flap. A contralateral pedicle also results in less visual obstruction. However, either if additional length is required for more caudal defects or if a shorter pedicle length is desired for patients with a lower hairline, an ipsilateral pedicle may be the design of choice.

Once again, pedicle length must be sufficient to ensure that the flap can reach the defect without tension. Additional length can be obtained by dissecting through the corrugator muscle and extending the pedicle into the brow and lower glabella. Periosteum can be incorporated with the flap at the base of the pedicle for more length and rigidity. As the pedicle base drifts more inferiorly, it can end up inferior to the supratrochlear notch and thus no longer incorporate that named vessel. Despite this modified design, the flap continues to be reliable and well perfused, suggesting that a major contributor to viability is the collateral flow and robust perfusion pressure to the subdermal plexus. This observation is further supported by previous studies demonstrating the presence of a robust anastomotic network of vessels within the glabella[7] (**Fig. 4**), permitting the effective use of a midline forehead flap in nasal reconstruction in which inclusion of the supratrochlear artery was not ensured.[18]

## PLANE OF ELEVATION

The distal aspect of the flap is usually elevated in the subcutaneous plane, leaving the frontalis and galea down on the forehead for the first third of the skin paddle, after which elevation continues in the subgaleal plane (**Fig. 5**). This proximal portion of the skin paddle will be thinned and debulked during pedicle division about 3 weeks later. Of note, some favor raising the entirety of the flap in the subgaleal plane because of less

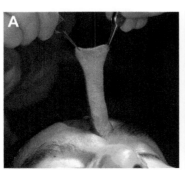
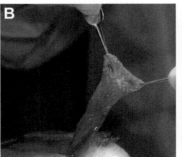
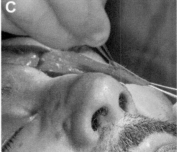

**Fig. 5.** Distal aspect of the flap is usually *elevated thin*, in the subcutaneous plane, to facilitate more effective flap thinning. (*A*) forehead flap elevated with narrow pedicle. (*B, C*) Flap after aggressive thinning of the distal aspect to match the thin skin of the alar lobule.

bleeding, and the flap can be thinned after elevation. Furthermore, primary closure would eventually require excision of the frontalis. We favor initially raising in the subcutaneous plane to facilitate more effective flap thinning. Should the donor site be wide and unable to close primarily, the optimal plan is to allow it to heal by second intent. Leaving the galea down at the primary stage will significantly accelerate the reepithelialization and contracture of this donor site. Smokers and other high-risk individuals undergoing planned 3-stage repair pose an exception. For these individuals, flap elevation incorporates the frontalis muscle and thinning is undertaken at the intermediate stage, 3 weeks after transposition.

## FLAP INSET

Before inset of the flap into the defect, the inferior border of the flap must be perfectly seated within the defect and free of gaps to prevent any vertical tension, which may result in cephalic retraction of the alar lobule, alar notching, and alar base asymmetry (**Fig. 6**). The edges should be beveled for

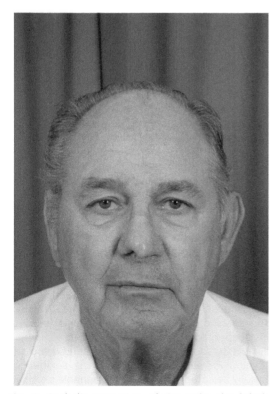

**Fig. 6.** Cephalic retraction of the right alar lobule. This can be prevented by ensuring that the inferior border of the flap is perfectly seated within the defect.

eversion. Additional aggressive thinning of the flap should be performed to match the intrinsic variations in native skin thickness for healthy patients. The native nasal skin is typically thick at the tip and nasion, and thin at the rhinion, columella, and alar rim.[19,20] The flap corresponding to the rhinion, columella, and alar rim should therefore be selectively thinned in healthy patients to the subdermal layer. Thinning should proceed around the axial subdermal vessels encountered within the galea without sacrificing the vessels. This step is deferred for smokers and other high-risk patients until the intermediate stage. Through-and-through quilting sutures can be used to restore nasal contour in key areas such as the supra-alar crease.

## DONOR SITE CLOSURE

Primary closure of donor site defects less than 3.5 cm wide can be typically achieved through wide undermining in the subgaleal plane out to the temples bilaterally. Deep sutures must be through the galeal layer for sufficient strength of closure. All deep sutures are typically placed before tying of sutures, allowing the suture needles to be accurately placed through the galea. The standing cutaneous deformity and the superior border are excised in a vertical fashion, with the incision extending superiorly past the hairline. Alternatively, O-to-T closure can be used, elevating bilateral subgaleal advancement flaps with a horizontal limb at the hairline. A W-plasty can be used to further camouflage the scar, with the hairline incision beveled opposite the direction of the hair follicles to allow hair growth through the scar.[21]

For any remaining defect that cannot be closed primarily, typically in the superior aspect of the forehead, healing by second intent usually yields optimal results (**Fig. 7**). For these patients, leaving the frontalis down on the donor site facilitates more rapid reepithelialization.

The application of expanded forehead flaps whereby tissue expanders are used before flap inset to reduce wound tension have previously been described.[22] Although expanded forehead flaps are thought to be favorable for avoiding hypertrophic scars and keloids in patients with higher Fitzpatrick skin types, it requires yet another operative stage after which the patient is subject to significant cosmetic deformity for an interval of time. The expanded skin is less favorable in terms of flap physiology, and some flap contracture will occur, compromising the final nasal form. For these reasons, tissue expansion is very rarely used in nasal reconstruction.

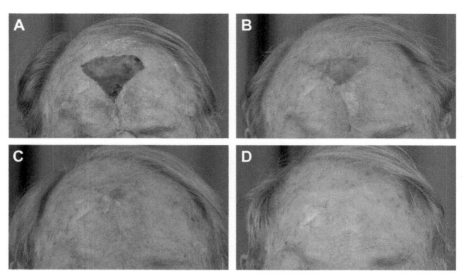

**Fig. 7.** Healing of donor site by second intent. (*A*) Two weeks after reconstruction. (*B*) Eight weeks after reconstruction. (*C*) Three months after reconstruction. (*D*) Nine months after reconstruction.

## THREE-STAGED FOREHEAD FLAP

Smokers, patients with a history of earlier radiation, patients with diabetes mellitus, and other patients with small vessel disease are at higher risk of partial necrosis and require a skin paddle with a more robust blood supply. In these populations, a 3-stage reconstructive approach is often used.[23,24] The addition of an intermediate stage allows for deferral of the thinning step often undertaken at the first stage for healthy patients. In the 3-stage approach, the first stage involves a complete subgaleal dissection throughout the skin paddle without thinning. After a 3-week interval, the frontalis muscle is debulked during the intermediate stage and selective flap thinning occurs. Cartilage grafts can be placed at this time. The final stage of standard pedicle division occurs 3 weeks afterward. Proponents of the 3-stage approach argue that it improves flap perfusion, expands lining and structural support options, and provides superior esthetic outcomes.[23,25]

## PEDICLE DIVISION

Pedicle division typically occurs approximately 3 weeks following initial flap inset to allow for adequate neovascularization of the flap from the underlying recipient tissue bed. This process may take longer depending on patient risk factors such as nicotine use and other comorbidities as well as defect properties such as size and depth. Before revascularization of the flap, the pedicle,

although posing significant cosmetic deformity, is the only nutrient source to the skin paddle.

The pedicle is first divided transversely a few millimeters above the original nasal defect (**Fig. 8**). This is followed by undermining immediately deep to the dermal plane, from a superior to inferior direction, continuing to halfway down the skin paddle. The subcutaneous tissue is then removed and the flap is debulked to conform to the normal nasal topography. The edges of the original nasal defects are freshened and corners squared off. The superior stump of the pedicle in the glabellar region is then trimmed and the corrugator muscle aggressively thinned before inset back into the glabella. There is a tendency for this small triangular flap to "pincushion" and leave a conspicuous contour irregularity. Great focus on reestablishing brow symmetry is paramount during this stage. This is accomplished by rotating the triangular flap superiorly and medially before inset, with the contralateral medial brow as the landmark. Many times, the inferior aspect of the vertical forehead closure can be revised at this time because it tends to heal with some inversion and widening. During this step, skin is excised but deeper scar should be left behind, when possible, to assist with scar support and eversion.

Timing for safe pedicle division is flexible. In carefully selected patients with amenable defects, it has been shown using laser-assisted indocyanine green angiography that it is possible to shorten this interval with division of the pedicle at 1 to 2 weeks after initial flap transfer.[26–28] For

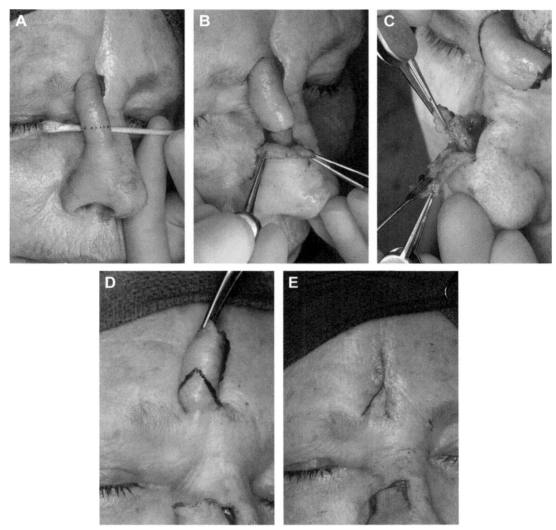

**Fig. 8.** Pedicle division. (*A*) Planned incision for pedicle division at the dotted line, a few millimeters above the original nasal defect. (*B*) The flap is undermined immediately deep to the dermal plane, from a superior to inferior direction, continuing to halfway down the skin paddle to the dotted line. (*C*) The subcutaneous tissue is removed and the flap is debulked to conform to the normal nasal topography. (*D*) The superior stump of the pedicle is then trimmed at the marked line and the corrugator muscle aggressively thinned before inset back into the glabella. (*E*) Triangular flap is inset with brow symmetry.

certain patient populations with defects limited to the upper two-thirds of the nose, it is possible to avoid pedicle division entirely by performing a *single-stage island forehead flap*, which uses a deep-ithelialized pedicle tunneled under intact glabellar skin[29,30] (**Fig. 9**). Usage of this flap should be avoided for defects of the nasal tip and ala, which require a lengthier forehead flap. The single-stage island forehead flap is supported by a unilateral supratrochlear artery and collateral supply from the angular artery. The flap should be based on the contralateral side to the defect to avoid excessive torsion on the pedicle. The glabellar skin is meticulously elevated and dissected off the pedicle with care taken to avoid changes in plane of dissection, which may result in pedicle amputation. Wide undermining of the glabellar skin is performed, and the tunnel is connected to the defect of the nose. Portions of the procerus muscle can be resected to prevent pedicle compression and congestion. The flap is tunneled under intact glabellar skin and inset into the nasal defect.

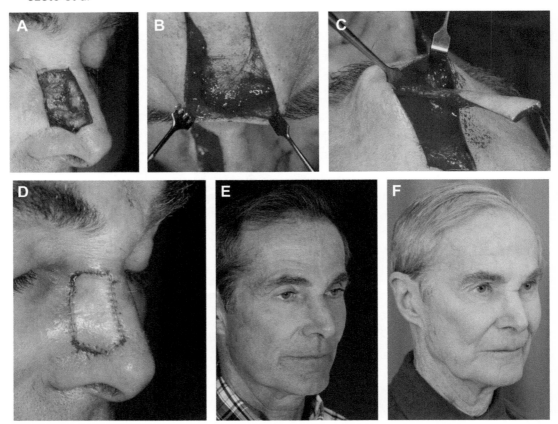

**Fig. 9.** Single-stage island forehead flap. (*A*) Right nasal sidewall defect limited to the upper two-thirds of the nose. (*B*) The pedicle is deepithelialized without compromising the vascular supply. (*C*) Wide undermining of the glabellar skin is performed to create a tunnel. (*D*) The flap is tunneled under intact glabellar skin and inset into the nasal defect. (*E*) Nine months following nasal reconstruction. (*F*) Twenty-two years after reconstruction.

## SUMMARY

The forehead flap is a reliable tool and provides predictable long-term results for resurfacing of large nasal defects. It can address all 3 separate layers of the nose in a full-thickness defect while providing a durable covering that is of similar thickness and texture to the native nasal skin. The various nuances of this technique discussed in this article are the guiding principles for forehead flap reconstruction of large nasal defects. These include the following:

1. Using a midline skin paddle for a more inconspicuous donor site scar.
2. Using a narrow pedicle contralateral to the defect for an improved arc of rotation without buckling of the blood supply.
3. Defect modification to ensure scars that are straight linear, with sharp corners and, whenever possible, in the midline of the nose. Final scars should not violate esthetic nasal subunit borders if possible.
4. Aggressive and selective thinning of the skin paddle to conform to native nasal topography.

5. Various methods for donor site closure, including direct excision of standing cutaneous deformity, O-to-T plasty, W-plasty, and healing by second intent.
6. Scar reexcision and restoration of brow symmetry during pedicle division.

## CLINICS CARE POINTS

The various nuances of this technique discussed in this article are the guiding principles for forehead flap reconstruction of large nasal defects. These include the following:

- Using a midline skin paddle for a more inconspicuous donor site scar.

- Using a narrow pedicle contralateral to the defect for an improved arc of rotation without buckling of the blood supply.

- Defect modification to ensure scars that are straight linear, with sharp corners and, whenever possible, in the midline of the nose. Final scars should not violate esthetic nasal subunit borders if possible.

- Aggressive and selective thinning of the skin paddle to conform to native nasal topography.
- Various methods for donor site closure, including direct excision of standing cutaneous deformity, O-to-T plasty, W-plasty, and healing by second intent.
- Scar reexcision and restoration of brow symmetry during pedicle division.

## DISCLOSURE

The authors have nothing to disclose.

## REFERENCES

1. Correa BJ, Weathers WM, Wolfswinkel EM, et al. The forehead flap: the gold standard of nasal soft tissue reconstruction. Semin Plast Surg 2013;27(2):96–103.
2. Zelken JA, Chang CS, Reddy SK, et al. Double forehead flap reconstruction of composite nasal defects. J Plast Reconstr Aesthetic Surg 2016;69(9):1280–4.
3. Burget GC, Menick FJ. The subunit principle in nasal reconstruction. Plast Reconstr Surg 1985;76(2):239–47.
4. Park SS. The flaring suture to augment the repair of the dysfunctional nasal valve. Plast Reconstr Surg 1998;101(4):1120–2.
5. Park SS. Reconstruction of nasal defects larger than 1.5 centimeters in diameter. Laryngoscope 2000;110(8):1241–50.
6. Kleintjes WG. Forehead anatomy: arterial variations and venous link of the midline forehead flap. J Plast Reconstr Aesthetic Surg 2007;60(6):593–606.
7. Reece EM, Schaverien M, Rohrich RJ. The paramedian forehead flap: a dynamic anatomical vascular study verifying safety and clinical implications. Plast Reconstr Surg 2008;121(6):1956–63.
8. Kazanjian VH, Roopenian A. Median forehead flaps in the repair of defects of the nose and surrounding areas. Trans Am Acad Ophthalmol Otolaryngol 1956;60(4):557–66.
9. Millard DR Jr. Total reconsttirucve rhinoplasty and a missing link. Plast Reconstr Surg 1966;37(3):167–83.
10. Millard DR Jr. Hemirhinoplasty. Plast Reconstr Surg 1967;40(5):440–5.
11. Millard DR Jr. Reconstructive rhinoplasty for the lower half of a nose. Plast Reconstr Surg 1974;53(2):133–9.
12. Millard DR Jr. Reconstructive rhinoplasty for the lower two-thirds of the nose. Plast Reconstr Surg 1976;57(6):722–8.
13. Yu D, Weng R, Wang H, et al. Anatomical study of forehead flap with its pedicle based on cutaneous branch of supratrochlear artery and its application in nasal reconstruction. Ann Plast Surg 2010;65(2):183–7.
14. Yen CI, Chang CJ, Chang CS, et al. Laser hair removal following forehead flap for nasal reconstruction. Laser Med Sci 2020;35(7):1549–54.
15. Tardy ME Jr, Sykes J, Kron T. The precise midline forehead flap in reconstruction of the nose. Clin Plast Surg 1985;12(3):481–94.
16. Menick FJ. Aesthetic refinements in use of forehead for nasal reconstruction: the paramedian forehead flap. Clin Plast Surg 1990;17(4):607–22.
17. Faris C, van der Eerden P, Vuyk H. The midline central artery forehead flap: a valid alternative to supratrochlear-based forehead flaps. JAMA Facial Plast Surg 2015;17(1):16–22.
18. Stigall LE, Bramlette TB, Zitelli JA, et al. The para-midline forehead flap: a clinical and microanatomic study. Dermatol Surg 2016;42(6):764–71.
19. Cho GS, Kim JH, Yeo NK, et al. Nasal skin thickness measured using computed tomography and its effect on tip surgery outcomes. Otolaryngol Head Neck Surg 2011;144(4):522–7.
20. Dey JK, Recker CA, Olson MD, et al. Assessing nasal soft-tissue envelope thickness for rhinoplasty: normative data and a predictive algorithm. JAMA Facial Plast Surg 2019;21(6):511–7.
21. Quatela VC, Sherris DA, Rounds MF. Esthetic refinements in forehead flap nasal reconstruction. Arch Otolaryngol Head Neck Surg 1995;121(10):1106–13.
22. Wei M, Bu X, Wang G, et al. Expanded forehead flap in Asian nasal reconstruction. Sci Rep 2023;13(1):5496.
23. Oleck NC, Hernandez JA, Cason RW, et al. Two or three? approaches to staging of the paramedian forehead flap for nasal reconstruction. Plast Reconstr Surg Glob Open 2021;9(5):e3591.
24. Menick FJ. A 10-year experience in nasal reconstruction with the three-stage forehead flap. Plast Reconstr Surg 2002;109(6):1839–55. discussion 1856-1861.
25. Jellinek NJ, Nguyen TH, Albertini JG. Paramedian forehead flap: advances, procedural nuances, and variations in technique. Dermatol Surg 2014;40(Suppl 9):S30–42.
26. Rudy SF, Abdelwahab M, Kandathil CK, et al. Paramedian forehead flap pedicle division after 7 days using laser-assisted indocyanine green angiography. J Plast Reconstr Aesthetic Surg 2021;74(1):116–22.
27. Calloway HE, Moubayed SP, Most SP. Cost-effectiveness of early division of the forehead flap pedicle. JAMA Facial Plast Surg 2017;19(5):418–20.
28. Shaye DA, Tollefson TT. What Is the Optimal Timing for Dividing a Forehead Flap? Laryngoscope 2020;130(10):2303–4.
29. Park SS. The single-stage forehead flap in nasal reconstruction: an alternative with advantages. Arch Facial Plast Surg 2002;4(1):32–6.
30. Fudem GM, Montilla RD, Vaughn CJ. Single-stage forehead flap in nasal reconstruction. Ann Plast Surg 2010;64(5):645–8.

# Revision Nasal Reconstruction After Previous Forehead Flap

Jeffrey Mella, MD, Samuel L. Oyer, MD*

## KEYWORDS

• Nasal defects • Failed nasal reconstruction • Revision nasal reconstruction • Revision forehead flap

## KEY POINTS

• Most major nasal reconstructions require multiple stages and many benefit from revisions to refine esthetics and function.
• Minor refinements are often accomplished with a single-stage outpatient procedure around 4 to 6 months after pedicle division.
• When minor revisions are inadequate, the primary reconstruction must be entirely redone with a second forehead flap.
• Priority must be given to both inner lining and structural support to optimize outcomes.
• A meticulously-planned multistage approach is recommended to properly execute a comprehensive reconstruction while allowing flexibility to perform adjustments along the way for any unforeseen healing issues.

## BACKGROUND/INTRODUCTION

Nasal reconstruction requires mastery of esthetic and surgical techniques to create a functionally stable and visually inconspicuous nose. With its central position on the face, nasal deformities infer a large social penalty to patients and significantly reduce their quality of life. Although "filling a defect" may seem straightforward, reconstructing a nose with the correct dimension, projection, structural support, symmetry, skin color, three-dimensional (3D) contour, and open airways is a challenging pursuit to even the most experienced surgeons. Most major nasal reconstructions require multiple stages, and many benefit from later revisions to refine esthetics and function. The forehead flap, with its origins in antiquity, remains the major workhorse for large or complex nasal defects and the gold standard for major nasal reconstruction.[1,2] This article highlights pitfalls and pearls for approaching revision nasal reconstruction following a prior forehead flap.

## PREDICTING REVISIONS

Minor revisions in nasal reconstruction are common and even predictable.[2,3] Appropriate preoperative counseling is essential so patients understand that these revisions are an opportunity for fine-tuning the result rather than correcting a failure.[4] Careful analysis of the defect with an eye to the future will elucidate possible refinements needed down the road. Educating patients about the anticipated potential revisions improves patient buy-in, especially when recommending a multistage approach. Harmony between the goals and expectations of surgeon and patient at the outset is required and supplies the needed long-term perspective for patients navigating the sometimes months long journey of complex nasal reconstruction. An accurate assessment of the risk of complications is also an essential component of the initial consultation. The site, size, and depth of the defect will determine the complexity of the repair and infer a greater likelihood for the

Department of Otolaryngology–Head and Neck Surgery, University of Virginia, Charlottesville, VA, USA
* UVA Department of Otolaryngology- Head and Neck Surgery, University of Virginia Health System, 1 Hospital Drive, PO Box 800713, Charlottesville, VA 22908.
E-mail address: SLO5FA@uvahealth.org

Facial Plast Surg Clin N Am 32 (2024) 281–289
https://doi.org/10.1016/j.fsc.2023.12.003

possibility of revision surgery. Potential for cancer recurrence, active smoking, autoimmune disease, vascular disease, prior radiation, or uncontrolled diabetes carry intuitive risk for complications and should be fully understood by both patient and surgeon.[3,4]

Initial surgical planning, meticulous template formation, and thoughtful application of nasal reconstructive principles are paramount and will set the course for a successful reconstruction. Even with precision planning and near perfect technical execution, complications may arise given the complexity of the task and limited margin for error. When such complications arise, prompt attention is critical to preserve as much of the reconstruction as possible. When unforeseen road bumps occur, threatening the final outcome, a multistage approach affords the additional opportunity to recognize minor errors or miscalculations and use on-the-fly adjustments during subsequent stages.[4,5]

## MINOR REVISIONS

If the initial forehead flap reconstruction is performed appropriately, only minor revisions are needed to reach the goal of normal nasal function and complete esthetic acceptance.[4,6] Predictable deformities that often require minor touch-ups include blunting of the alar crease, excess width of the nostril margins with narrowed external nasal valves, or conspicuous donor site facial scars. Minor refinements are often accomplished with a single-stage outpatient procedure around 4 to 6 months after pedicle division.[3] Most minor deformities are amenable to correction with direct incisions falling between nasal subunits to recreate natural creases, rather than using the location of the original incisions which may have been dictated more by the defect location than optimal nasal esthetics.[2,4] Soft tissue excisions or flap elevation to remove excess volume is best performed once the vascularity of a flap is ensured. Soft tissue sculpting or cartilage onlay grafting should be used to match the uninvolved side. Standard rhinoplasty maneuvers, such as tip refinement sutures, tip grafting, or camouflage grafting can be used to improve the overall symmetry and shape of the nose. Modifying the native nasal cartilage can improve the final outcome, even when that cartilage was not involved in the original nasal defect. Whenever possible, the patient's contralateral native nasal subunits should be used to create templates of the normal nasal subunits as an ideal guide for incision placement. When contralateral subunits are unavailable, preoperative photos are an invaluable resource.[5,6]

Asymmetry of the alar crease is a classic example of an anticipated deformity after reconstruction of a nasal ala and sidewall defect with a blunted crease on the reconstructed side. Following initial reconstruction, the crease can be improved through a separate incision along the desired location of the crease 3 to 6 months later. Excess underlying soft tissue and/or cartilage are sculpted into a depression mirroring the contralateral side and the skin is tacked down to accentuate the crease (Fig. 1A–E).

Notching of the nostril margin is a potential deformity following nasal reconstruction of defects involving the alar margin. Based on the size of the notch present, this revision should not be underestimated, as even a relatively small notch often requires a composite reconstruction of lining, structural support, and overlying skin to achieve a lasting result. Simply repairing one layer of skin in these cases is often fraught with reformation of the notch. Composite grafts taken from the ear are excellent for reconstructing a limited loss of inner lining with structural support and can be combined with a local transposition flap of external skin for vascularized coverage (Fig. 2A–F).

Excess width at the nostril margin is another frequently encountered imperfection and requires minor revisions to reestablish an acceptable nasal airway along with nostril symmetry. The ideal location of the nostril margin is identified based on a template of the contralateral nostril and incised along this junction. Nasal lining is elevated and soft tissue, mostly scar, is excised. The internal surface of previously placed cartilage grafts may be carefully shaved taking care to maintain their support and vascularity.[7] When lining deficits are encountered, small local transposition flaps can be developed from excessive nostril margin or columellar skin.

## MAJOR REVISIONS

When the goal of restoring a functionally intact and esthetically inconspicuous nose falls drastically short, a major revision is required. Whether the result of improper planning or serious complication, extensive distortions of nasal form and function may require significant revisions to the original reconstruction or often times require a complete redo with an entirely new nasal reconstruction.[7] Although it may seem daunting to the patient and the surgeon to undergo an entirely new series of surgeries, essentially repeating the reconstruction, attempts at multiple small interventions to shortcut a larger revision surgery often fail to achieve the desired results and could even further compromise the nasal form or function.

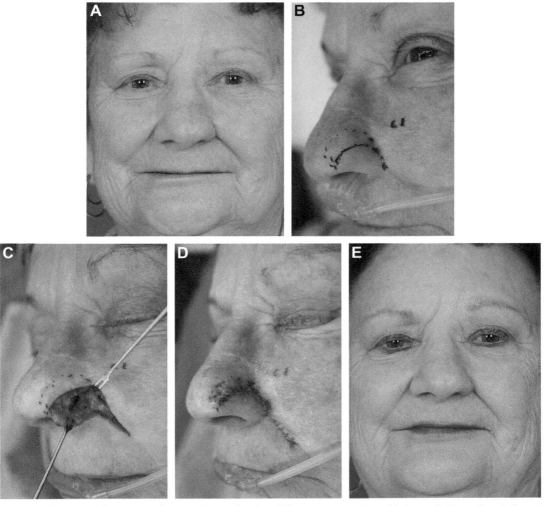

**Fig. 1.** (*A*) Three months post-op from a primary forehead flap reconstruction of left nasal sidewall and ala with predicted blunting of the left alar crease. (*B*) Six months after initial reconstruction, the revision is designed by marking the desired location of alar crease for the planned direct incision. (*C*) The skin is elevated and excess underlying soft tissue and/or cartilage are sculpted into a depression mirroring the contralateral side. (*D*) The incision is closed and tacking sutures above the alar crease are used to close the dead space created during sculpting. (*E*) Three months post-revision surgery with improved alar crease symmetry.

## PREOPERATIVE COUNSELING FOR A MAJOR REVISION

During the initial consultation for revision surgery, patient expectations must be thoroughly explored and understood. Frank discussions are warranted regarding the patient's desired outcome and their willingness to undergo another multistage reconstruction. First delineating whether the patient prefers to work with what they have to improve the original reconstruction, even if the result remains imperfect, or do they wish to "start over" with another multistage major reconstruction. Before recommending a revision major nasal reconstruction, it is worth pausing to consider the reasons for

inadequate primary repair. Are there identifiable reasons that the reconstruction went off the rails that can confidently be avoided this time around? An honest assessment of the surgeon's skills and the patient's medical fitness is critical before embarking on yet another round of major surgeries to ensure a realistic chance of success in offering the patient the improvement they are seeking. In the revision setting, patient expectations are often defined by prior experiences and may need significant adjustments to fit any anatomic or physiologic limitations that revision surgery entails. Even patients who've had a forehead flap in the past require a detailed understanding of the

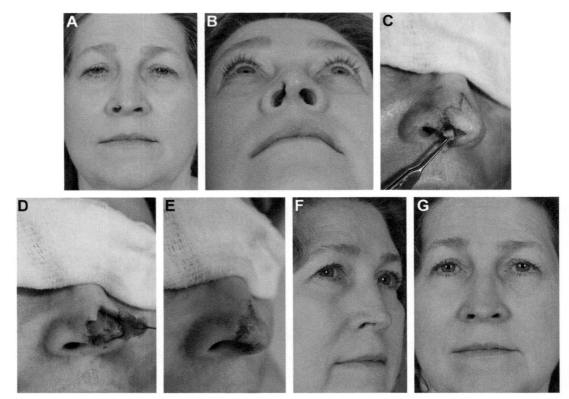

**Fig. 2.** (*A*) Frontal view demonstrating right alar notching following a previous nasal reconstruction. (*B*) Base view demonstrating right alar notching following a previous nasal reconstruction. (*C*) A minor revision is designed with an auricular composite graft to reconstruct the inner lining and provide the required support of the soft tissue triangle. (*D*) A bilobed flap designed, elevated, and transposed to reconstruct the external soft tissue and nourish the composite graft. This is designed to the primary lobe reaches around the desired alar rim to sew to the skin of the composite graft. (*E*) Oblique view of the closure demonstrating improved alar margin contour and resolution of notching. (*F*) Oblique view: 6 months post-revision surgery demonstrating improved alar margin contour and symmetry. (*G*) Frontal view: 6 months post-revision surgery demonstrating improved alar margin contour and symmetry.

logistical inconveniences associated with an interpolated flap pedicle and the extra scarring of the forehead. Before proceeding, the overall reconstructive strategy and anticipated timeline of the multiple stages must be completely understood by the motivated patient.

## SURGICAL PLANNING

When evaluating a reconstruction with esthetic imperfections, it is helpful to try and look at the nose globally, ignoring the prior reconstruction, to identify specific targets for further treatment. Using a consistent systematic approach to nasal analysis will ensure all priorities are accounted for. Evaluate the patient's old operative reports, postoperative course including any complications, and preoperative photographs to understand the defect that existed before the primary reconstruction. Which aspects of the defect were inadequately treated?

A sound surgical plan starts with an accurate list of the deficiencies that exist and the techniques required to address them. A precise understanding of the available donor tissue is paramount. What options exist for replacing nasal lining? Is septal or auricular cartilage available for structural grafting? Are vascular pedicles available for harvesting a second forehead flap? What is the laxity of the donor tissue and does it require tissue expansion? Regardless of the defect, when performing a major revision nasal reconstruction, a staged approach is highly recommended. A multistage reconstruction has invaluable advantages including the ability to recreate a true defect, build a stable support platform with cartilage grafting, improve flap survival with vascular delay, donor tissue expansion, prelamination, and perhaps most significantly to allow needed course corrections for any miscalculations or wound healing issues along the way.[7]

## INNER LINING

Inadequate replacement of nasal inner lining during the primary nasal reconstruction is frequently a common denominator among patients requiring a major revision and should be a priority while approaching revision surgery.[8] Finding donor tissue for nasal lining can be challenging but several options exist. If available, using "like-tissue" with available donor nasal lining is preferred. Such options include the inferior turbinate mucosal flap, a bipedicled "bucket-handle" mucosal flap, or nasoseptal composite flap. These options are often lacking adequate tissue to reconstruct a significant deficiency of nasal lining. A pericranial flap is a reliable source of thin and pliable vascularized tissue, but the vascularity may have been compromised with the initial reconstruction. One advantage to revision nasal reconstruction is that it often affords cutaneous tissue that would otherwise be discarded while recreating the defect or completion excision of nasal esthetic subunits.[5] In this setting, the *epithelial turn-in flap* provides a versatile option for internal defects of the middle and lower third of the nose. Care must be taken to elevate in the subdermal plane distally before transitioning to a deeper plane proximally to create a flap with a robust enough pedicle to withstand the 180° "turn-in." In situations where the survival of the flap is threatened due to patient comorbidities or prior radiation, a staged vascular delay procedure may be used to bolster the vascular supply of this flap through the subcutaneous pedicle (**Figs. 3**A–P and **4**A–D). The ideal defect for this type of a flap has the intranasal edge in close proximity to the cutaneous edge allowing for primary edge-to-edge approximation.[3,7]

## STRUCTURAL SUPPORT

Significant impairment in nasal airway function is a common complaint among patients seeking major revision following nasal reconstruction.[8] Inadequate bolstering of the lateral nasal wall with cartilage grafts frequently leads to both static and dynamic collapse of the internal and external nasal valves. Excess soft tissue bulk from internal or external reconstructive flaps can also impair nasal breathing. When inadequate consideration is given to reconstructing the internal nasal lining, long-term contracture can lead to circumferential vestibular stenosis. Thus, when approaching a revision nasal reconstruction, repeat contracture must be anticipated and planned for with appropriate attention given to structural support. Revision cases may benefit from "over-engineering" the structural support with strong cartilage grafting

when the cause of the initial failure was inadequate support.[9] Preoperative understanding of donor site availability for cartilage grafts guide decision-making. Careful consideration must be used to know whether soft malleable ear cartilage versus the stiffness or rigidity of costal cartilage is required. Costal cartilage, either autologous or cadaveric, is frequently required as a source of cartilage grafting in the revision setting when donor cartilage is limited. Cartilage can be harvested from the seventh, eighth, or ninth rib and include the bony cartilaginous junction if there is a defect of the bony nasal dorsum. When additional rigid structural support is needed along the upper one-third, a split calvarial bone can be harvested from the abundant straight parietal region of the skull. Structural grafts are often placed during the initial surgical stage with the transfer of a forehead flap or at an intermediate-stage procedure before pedicle division.[3,10,11]

## THE REVISION FOREHEAD FLAP

When minor revisions to a prior forehead flap nasal reconstruction are inadequate, the primary reconstruction must be entirely redone with a second forehead flap.[7] As detailed in other articles in this issue, the forehead flap is not strictly axial, so a second or even third forehead flap harvest is possible.[11,12] The first stage sets the course for the successful revision. The defect must be recreated to fully define the position and volume of tissue loss and the requirements of reconstruction, confirming what was suspected during the preoperative analysis. It is critical during this first stage to fully evaluate the primary reconstruction for opportunities for salvage by repurposing skin or prior cartilage grafts before discarding any tissue. If appropriate, epithelial turn-in flaps may be prepared with vascular delay (see **Fig. 4**D).

The donor site is then meticulously prepared for a second flap. The processes of biologic and mechanical creep along with the natural laxity of the forehead are usually adequate to allow harvesting a second forehead flap without tissue expansion.[12] However, in patients with minimal scalp laxity or limited non-hair-bearing forehead skin, a tissue expander may be inserted during the first stage and beginning at 3 weeks postoperatively, serially expanded for a total of 12 weeks to provide adequate donor skin.[13] Some argue that the post-tissue expander flap is more pliable and able to conform to the 3D shape of the nose, however, flap contraction is commonly seen following removal of the expander, so slightly oversizing the flap dimensions is recommended to account for this contraction. The successful forehead flap

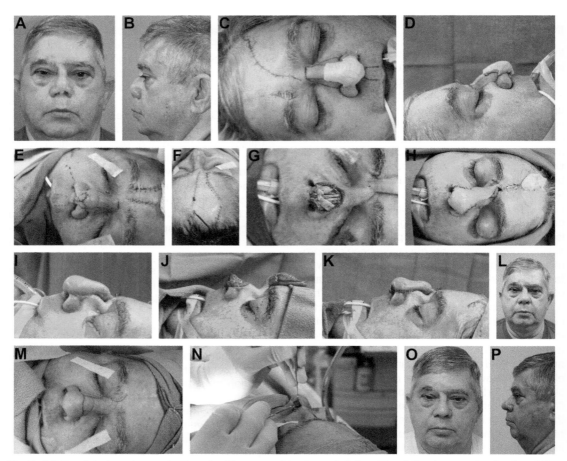

**Fig. 3.** (*A*) Frontal view demonstrating significant persistent nasal deformities following a prior forehead flap reconstruction with an undersized, contracted, and pincushioned appearance. (*B*) Profile view demonstrating the underprojected prior forehead flap reconstruction. (*C*) Frontal view: Surgical putty was used to form the overall desired dimensions of his nose. The template for the revision forehead flap was made from this appropriately sized nose. (*D*) Profile View: Surgical putty was used to form the overall desired dimensions of his nose. The template for the revision forehead flap was made from this appropriately sized nose. (*E*) Stage 1: Vascular delay was used to prepare columellar turn-in flaps. (*F*) Vascular delay was also used to prepare the left forehead flap to improve the predictability of the vascularity of this flap because the original flap used a right-sided pedicle and a left-sided skin paddle. (*G*) Stage 2: The defect was re-created and turn-in flaps rotated to create internal lining. Structural integrity of the reconstruction was achieved with grafting using cadaveric rib and auricular composite grafts of the soft-tissue triangles. (*H*) Stage 2. Right paramedian forehead flap transferred into place. Upper forehead defect allowed healing secondarily. (*I*) Stage 3. Profile view following second stage demonstrating improved nasal projection but significant bulkiness of the flap with mismatch in thickness between the flap and surrounding nasal skin. (*J*) Stage 3: The entire forehead flap is elevated back on its pedicle taking care to preserve the underlying cartilaginous framework. The flap is thinned and sculpted before insetting again. Modifications to the vascularized cartilage framework are possible at this time. (*K*) Profile view following Stage 3 demonstrating improvement in flap bulk and projection. (*L*) At 4 months post-op (following Stage 3), the patient was noted to have improved nasal dimensions but the flap was noted to be persistently bulky with thickened donor site scar. (*M*) A final revision 1 year following pedicle division included forehead scar revision, excision of thickened nasal scar, and elevation of the superior half of the flap with thinning. (*N*) A final revision 1 year following pedicle division included forehead scar revision, excision of thickened nasal scar, and elevation of the superior half of the flap with thinning. (*O*) Frontal view: Final result 1 year after revision forehead flap reconstruction. (*P*) Profile view: Final result 1 year after revision forehead flap reconstruction.

hinges on a precise and accurate template.[4,6] Flap design must be meticulous and based on the uninvolved side to define the ideal or normal. When no premorbid nasal subunits are available to serve as a template, preoperative photographs can guide the creation of a 3D putty that can provide the necessary template from which the surgeon can create a 2D design for flap harvest (see **Fig. 3**C,

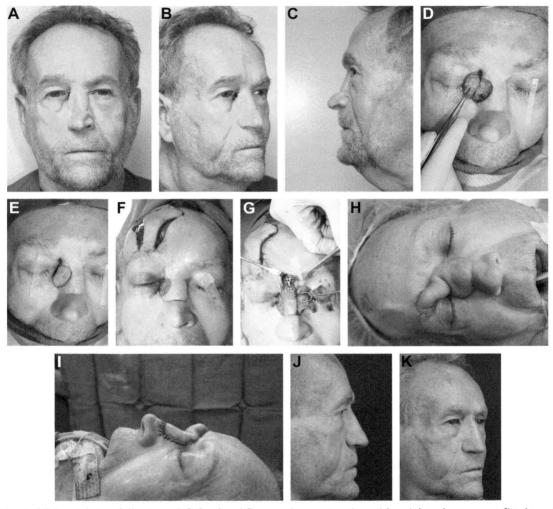

**Fig. 4.** (*A*) Frontal view following a left forehead flap nasal reconstruction with a right subcutaneous fistula and collapse of the nasal dorsum. Of note, the patient required postoperative radiotherapy following resection of his sinonasal malignancy. (*B*) Oblique view demonstrating the subcutaneous fistula adjacent to the right medial canthus. (*C*) Profile view demonstrating significant nasal dorsal collapse. (*D*) Stage 1: A medially based turn-in flap was designed to reconstruct the inner-lining for closure of the fistula. (*E*) Stage 1: Vascular delay was used to aid flap viability in a post-radiated field. (*F*) Stage 2: A second forehead flap was designed with a right supraorbital artery pedicle given the prior resection of the supratrochlear artery and prior left forehead flap. (*G*) Stage 2: An osseocartilaginous rib graft was used for structural support, restoring dorsal projection. (*H*) Stage 3: The subcutaneous fistula is closed. The still-pedicled forehead flap is thickened with significant height mismatch and bulk. (*I*) Stage 3: The forehead flap is left pedicled, elevated distally to improve contour, and re-inset. (*J*) Profile view: 3 months post-pedicle division with a healed subcutaneous fistula and improved dorsal projection. (*K*) Oblique view: 3 months post-pedicle division with a healed subcutaneous fistula and improved dorsal projection.

D). Printing of life-sized nasal models can also be performed based on a CT scan or 3D photo of the patient's nose before the initial insult, when these types of images are available.

If the prior forehead flap has compromised both supratrochlear arteries, an axial flap can be designed over the supraorbital artery (**Fig. 4**F). Consideration of pre-lamination or vascular delay before flap elevation is especially important in the

revision setting depending on the reason for initial reconstruction failure.[11] If the patient is willing to accept a conservative approach with multiple intermediate stages before pedicle division, this allows for aggressive flap elevation and exposure to fine-tune the soft tissue sculpting and structural grafting for a finesse approach. The multiple stages also provide opportunity for on-the-fly adjustments to unforeseen issues with graft or flap healing. Internal lining flaps are prone to contracture restenosis and may require stenting during the initial stages.[14,15]

Once the pedicle is divided, further touch-ups of the distal aspect of the flap should be delayed at least 4 months, likely longer in the revision setting, to avoid compromising the vascularity and viability of the structural grafts and overlying flap. The surgeon should not underestimate the power of allowing time for natural healing, particularly when waiting for edema of the flap to subside. Special care should be taken, however, to identify issues that led to the initial reconstructive failure and potential opportunities to intervene early when needed. Close follow-up and thorough patient communication during the healing process is paramount to a successful revision nasal reconstruction.[16,17]

## CASE PRESENTATIONS
### Case 1

A 63-year-old man presented after undergoing a prior left-sided oblique forehead flap for a full-thickness nasal tip defect. The flap was undersized without appropriate reconstruction of the internal lining or cartilaginous framework resulting in a fore-shortened and truncated appearance and right side nasal obstruction. During stage 1, vascular delay was used to prepare the left forehead flap and columellar turn-in flaps. The delay of the forehead flap was used to improve the predictability of the vascularity of this flap because the original flap used a right-sided pedicle and a left-sided skin paddle. Stage 2 included recreating the defect, folding and securing the columellar turn-in flaps, structural grafting with cadaveric rib and auricular composite grafts, and right paramedian forehead flap transfer. Optimal sizing of the reconstructed nose can be difficult in these cases where there is not an available remaining subunit to serve as a template. In this case, surgical putty was used to form the overall desired dimensions of his nose based on surrounding facial features, and the template for the forehead flap was made from this appropriately sized nose. In his third stage, the pedicle was divided, and the flap was elevated, thinned, and replaced at the brow. At 4 months, the patient was noted to have improved nasal dimension but the flap was noted to be bulky with thickened scar. A final revision 1 year following pedicle division included forehead scar revision, excision of thickened nasal scar, and elevation of the superior half of the flap with thinning (see **Fig. 3**A–P).

### Case 2

A 65-year-old man underwent prior resection of sinonasal squamous cell carcinoma of the midline nasal dorsum extending into the right anterior ethmoid sinus and abutting the orbit and skull base. His initial reconstruction included a left paramedian forehead flap, radial forearm flap for maxillary reconstruction, and orbital plating for the medial orbital wall and floor. The patient required postoperative radiotherapy complicated by the development of a right sinocutaneous fistula medial to the right medial canthus. In addition, a significant loss of dorsal projection and support occurred as seen on profile view.

The patient was counseled about options and elected to undergo a three-stage revision forehead flap reconstruction. The first stage involved a vascular delay of a right lateral nasal wall cutaneous turn-in flap (see **Fig. 2**). His second stage included the turn-in flap to recreate internal lining and excision of the old paramedian forehead flap (PMFF) skin to recreate the nasal defect. An osseocartilaginous rib graft was used to restore the dorsal nasal support securing this to the frontal bone with a mini plate. The skin defect was resurfaced with a forehead flap centered over the right supraorbital artery as the supratrochlear artery and associated frontal bone had been resected with the tumor. At 1-year follow-up, the patient is seen with a closed sinocutaneous fistula, improvement in his nasal profile, and an overall esthetically acceptable and functionally intact nose (**Fig. 4**A–K).

## SUMMARY

Nasal reconstruction is fraught with challenges for even the most experienced surgeons. Most major nasal reconstructions require late revisions to address persistent disruptions in form or function and this should be discussed with the patient before starting the reconstructive process. Minor revisions are often predictable and usually amenable to direct incisions placed between nasal subunits and soft tissue sculpting or augmentation with structural grafting. When minor revisions are inadequate, the initial reconstruction must be redone with a revision major nasal reconstruction. Harmony between patient and surgeon regarding expectations for outcomes and the realities of what is required is essential. A meticulously-planned multistage approach is invaluable to properly execute a comprehensive reconstruction while allowing for unforeseen needed adjustments along the way.

## CLINICS CARE POINTS

- Most major nasal reconstructions require multiple stages and many benefit from revisions to refine esthetics and function.

- When performing a major revision nasal reconstruction, priority must be given to inner lining and structural support to optimize the final outcome.
- The epithelial turn-in flap is particularly useful in the revision setting and provides a versatile option for inner lining defects by repurposing skin from the prior reconstruction.
- A multistage approach allows for aggressive flap elevation for soft tissue sculpting for a finesse apporach and provides opportunity for on the fly adjustments to address unanticipated issues.

## DISCLOSURE

The authors have no financial disclosures.

## REFERENCES

1. Correa BJ, Weathers WM, Wolfswinkel EM, et al. The forehead flap: the gold standard of nasal soft tissue reconstruction. Semin Plast Surg 2013;27(2): 96–103.
2. Menick FJ. Aesthetic refinements in use of forehead for nasal reconstruction: the paramedian forehead flap. Clin Plast Surg 1990;17(4):607–22.
3. Rosen CA. Bailey's head and neck surgery: otolaryngology. Philadelphia, PA: Lippincott Williams & Wilkins; 2022.
4. Quatela VC, Sherris DA, Rounds MF. Esthetic refinements in forehead flap nasal reconstruction. Arch Otolaryngol Head Neck Surg 1995;121(10): 1106–13.
5. Burget GC, Menick FJ. The subunit principle in nasal reconstruction. Plast Reconstr Surg 1985;76(2): 239–47.
6. Park SS. Reconstruction of nasal defects larger than 1.5 centimeters in diameter. Laryngoscope 2000; 110(8):1241–50.
7. Menick FJ. Revising or redoing an imperfect or failed nasal reconstruction. Facial Plast Surg 2014; 342–56.
8. Chen CL, Most SP, Branham GH, et al. Postoperative complications of paramedian forehead flap reconstruction. JAMA facial plastic surgery 2019;21(4): 298–304.
9. Austin GK, Shockley WW. Reconstruction of nasal defects: contemporary approaches. Curr Opin Otolaryngol Head Neck Surg 2016;453.
10. Millard DR Jr. Total reconstructive rhinoplasty and a missing link. Plast Reconstr Surg 1966;37(3): 167–83.
11. Ziegler JP, Oyer SL. Prelaminated paramedian forehead flap for subtotal nasal reconstruction using three-dimensional printing. BMJ Case Reports CP 2021;e238146.
12. Zelken JA, Chang CS, Reddy SK, et al. Double forehead flap reconstruction of composite nasal defects. J Plast Reconstr Aesthetic Surg 2016;69(9):1280–4.
13. Kheradmand Ali A. Ata Garajei, and Mohammad Hosein Kalantar Motamedi. "Nasal reconstruction: experience using tissue expansion and forehead flap". J Oral Maxillofac Surg 2011;69(5):1478–84.
14. Menick FJ. A 10-year experience in nasal reconstruction with the three-stage forehead flap. Plast Reconstr Surg 2002;109(6):1839–55 [discussion: 1856-1861].
15. Oleck NC, Hernandez JA, Cason RW, et al. Two or Three? Approaches to Staging of the Paramedian Forehead Flap for Nasal Reconstruction. Plast Reconstr Surg Glob Open 2021;9(5):e3591.
16. Menick FJ. Practical details of nasal reconstruction. Plast Reconstr Surg 2013;131(4):613e–30e.
17. Menick FJ. An approach to the late revision of a failed nasal reconstruction. Plast Reconstr Surg 2012;129(1):92e–103e.

# Reconstruction of Large Composite Defects Extending Beyond the Nose

Dominic Vernon, MD[a],*, Taha Z. Shipchandler, MD[b]

## KEYWORDS

- Nasal reconstruction • Composite defect • Forehead flap

## KEY POINTS

- Composite nasal defects should be categorized into the involved facial units.
- Use separate flaps/surgical plans for each involved facial unit.
- Establish a stable midface platform before nasal reconstruction.
- Staged nasal repair should be considered for larger composite defects.

## INTRODUCTION

Navigating the composite nasal defect requires attention to detail, meticulous planning, and patience. Multiple factors are at play when managing these complex reconstructions. In addition to addressing concerns related to nasal inner lining, structural support, and cutaneous coverage, the surgeon must also consider other involved facial subunits, additional risk for scar contracture, and loss of tissues supporting the nasal base. Planning should carefully identify the involved facial structures. Often, tissues comprising a stable base for the nose will need to be reconstructed before proceeding with the nasal reconstruction. As such, patience is key to an esthetically pleasing result, and patients should be counseled regarding the needs for multiple-staged surgeries. This article will address surgical planning and approaches for these large complex composite nasal defects.

## DEFINING INVOLVED FACIAL UNITS

Just as a defect that is isolated to the nose, large composite defects should be approached systematically. For nearly 40 years now, facial reconstructive surgeons have adhered to Burget's and Menick's nasal subunit principle when approaching

nasal reconstruction.[1] Scars are hidden within subunit borders when possible, and defects involving more than half of a subunit are often enlarged and completely resurfaced. Every effort is made to replace skin with new tissue that is of similar color, thickness, and texture.

Similar principles, with a few additions, can be applied to more complicated composite nasal defects. The defect must be characterized not only by the involved nasal subunits but also by the facial units involved. Naturally, the adjacent units are those typically involved, including the cheeks, upper lip, and medial canthal areas. In planning for surgery, it is helpful to delineate which of these units will need reconstructed. With unilateral defects, the contralateral facial unit serves as an excellent template for determining the amount of tissue loss and optimally restoring symmetry.

Only after the defect and its involved units are established should the surgeon design a surgical plan. A key point in large composite defects is that, when possible, different facial units should be reconstructed with separate flaps or surgical approaches. In the modern era of free tissue transfer, it is often easier to use a single flap to resurface or fill a large composite defect with healthy vascularized tissue. However, although this "fills the hole" and addresses the wound, it results in an

[a] Indiana University School of Medicine, 1115 Ronald Reagan Parkway, Suite 254, Avon, IN 46123, USA;
[b] Indiana University School of Medicine, 11725 Illinois Street, Suite 275, Carmel, IN 46032, USA
* Corresponding author.
E-mail address: dovernon@iupui.edu

Facial Plast Surg Clin N Am 32 (2024) 291–302
https://doi.org/10.1016/j.fsc.2024.01.006
1064-7406/24/© 2024 Elsevier Inc. All rights reserved.

amorphous appearance without any defined facial subunits. It also replaces facial skin with skin that is a poor match in color and texture. Whenever feasible, surgeons should attempt to reconstruct "like with like" and use local flaps even for complicated facial defects.[2] Exceptions obviously exist regarding this guideline; at times, there is simply not enough local tissue to accomplish this task and free flaps may be necessary for either bulk or to resurface a very large skin defect.

## IMPORTANCE OF WOUND DEPTH

Symmetry is an integral part of a successful nasal reconstruction. The nose rests on a platform of tissue composed of the maxilla, premaxillary tissues, and the skin and subcutaneous tissues of the bilateral cheeks and upper lip. Failure to recognize and account for a deficiency of tissue in any of these areas can result in an unstable base for nasal reconstruction. Subsequent scarring and contraction can thus have a detrimental effect on the repair, distorting any attempted nasal reconstruction, particularly in the alar region.

Assessing the depth and volume of tissue loss is crucial to both the timing and type of repair. Smaller composite defects limited to skin may be considered for concurrent repair of the nose and involved facial unit. Great care must still be taken in such circumstances to prevent distortion of the nasal tissues as the surrounding tissue contracts and heals. In general, surgeons should have a low threshold to stage larger composite defects, particularly those with a loss of deeper tissues of the cheek or premaxillary regions. A stable midface platform should be constructed before proceeding with nasal reconstruction in such cases.[2–4] Patients should be counseled regarding the need for multiple procedures.

Given the need for staged procedures, familiarity with the prelaminated forehead flap technique can be of great use in composite defects involving full thickness defects of the nose. The forehead flap can be raised, surfaced with a skin graft, and inset back into the forehead during the initial cheek or lip reconstruction.[5] The prelaminated graft is thus ready for nasal reconstruction by the time healing from the first stage is complete.

## APPROACH TO THE DEFECT
### Addressing Concurrent Cheek Defects

Large nasal defects frequently encroach on the medial cheek. As mentioned previously, the most successful results will be those that separately address the nose and the cheek defects. For cheek defects involving only skin, a simultaneous

repair can be considered (**Figs. 1–3**). Cervicofacial flaps work well to advance skin medially and reestablish the nasofacial sulcus, hiding the incisions between the nasal and cheek facial units.[6,7] The flap should be secured to periosteum of the medial maxilla or nasal bones to prevent contracture.

For deeper defects, efforts should be made to restore the lost volume over the piriform aperture, and greater consideration should be given to staging the nasal repair. For defects involving more subcutaneous tissue at the piriform, a medially-based subcutaneous hinge flap can often be used to restore volume, followed by resurfacing with skin advancement flaps.[4] If the resection includes all soft tissues down to the level of the maxilla, this may be insufficient. In such cases, if there is sufficient lateral cheek tissue remaining, an superficial musculoaponeurotic system (SMAS) flap can be mobilized from the free medial edge and recruited to fill the deficient tissue over the medial maxilla and piriform. Drilling holes in the maxilla for placement of sutures to secure the SMAS flap is often required if periosteum is absent.

Bony defects, if present, must be reconstructed before the soft tissues.[3] For less-extensive defects, free calvarial or iliac bone grafts work well.[4] Free tissue transfer, discussed later, can be considered for large bony and soft tissue defects.

### Addressing Concurrent Lip Defects

As with cheek defects, concurrent lip defects in composite nasal reconstruction should be thought of as distinct defect with a reconstructive plan that is separate, and often staged, from the nasal reconstruction. In composite nasal defects, it is the upper lip that warrants the most discussion. A complete review of upper lip reconstruction is beyond the scope of this article but its context in the setting of composite nasal reconstruction should focus on rebuilding subunits. Recall that the upper lip is more complex than the lower, and that the cutaneous white lip consists of the central philtrum and left and right cutaneous upper lip. Care should be taken to design incisions and scars to lie along the borders of these units whenever possible. The depth of the wound will determine whether a concurrent or staged approach should be undertaken. Regardless, separately reconstructing the nose and the lip will best restore the alar groove and prevent a blunted appearance to this facial landmark.

Cutaneous lateral lip defects can often be reconstructed with a V-Y advancement flap, advancing tissues to the alar groove. For smaller full thickness defects, bilateral advancement flaps

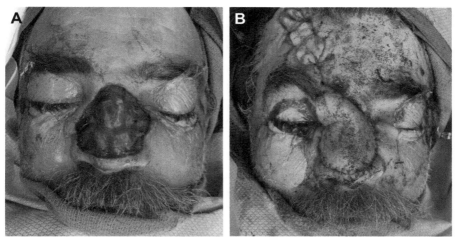

**Fig. 1.** Superficial composite defect. This large cutaneous nasal defect encroaches on bilateral cheek tissues. (*A*) Failure to recognize this will result in effacement of the nasofacial sulcus. Small bilateral cheek advancement flaps were made and secured to the periosteum of the nasal bones and maxilla. This sets the nasofacial sulcus before insetting of the forehead flap. (*B*) This composite defect involved skin only and concurrent cheek and nasal reconstruction was performed.

work well. However, if the philtrum is present, a lower threshold should exist to choose other options to avoid distortion of the philtral columns from advancement flaps. Abbe flaps work very well with more lateral full thickness defects because the incisions can be designed to lie on the border of the philtrum and avoid excessive tension on this central structure.[8]

Composite nasal defects of the nose and upper lip will frequently require resurfacing of the nasal sill and floor. Careful planning can often use the lip reconstruction to resurface this area concurrently. Advancement flaps frequently involve excision of standing cutaneous deformities lateral to the alar rim; these tissues can instead be left intact with the flap and rotated medially to resurface the nasal floor.[8] Similarly, an extended Abbe flap can resurface the nasal sill and floor during the first stage of composite reconstruction (**Figs. 4** and **5**). Similar to cheek reconstruction, more complex or

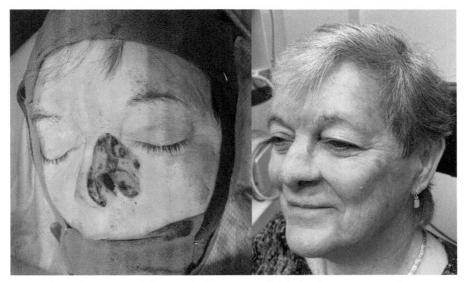

**Fig. 2.** Large near-hemirhinectomy defect, including a superficial cheek component. Concurrent repair with cheek advancement flap at time of first stage paramedian repair was performed. Three-quarter postoperative view on right.

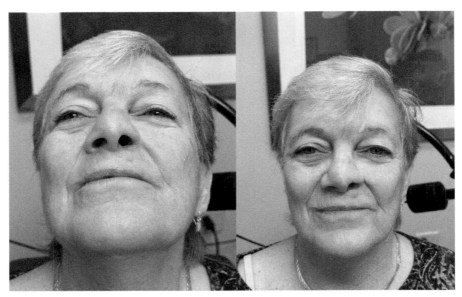

**Fig. 3.** Base and frontal view, 2-year postoperative photos of patient from **Fig. 2**.

larger upper lip defects should be addressed first, before proceeding with the nasal repair.

### Addressing the Medial Canthal Region

Large nasal defects may involve the medial canthal region, and surgeons should be familiar with and prepared to reconstruct this area. In general, smaller defects without eyelid involvement heal favorably, whereas defects involving the eyelids require more careful planning. The lower lid is more likely to be involved for resections originating from a nasal malignancy.

An isolated medial canthal defect without eyelid involvement is a concave area that heals favorably with little reconstruction. Although more complicated island or rotational flaps have been described, often the simple placement of a full

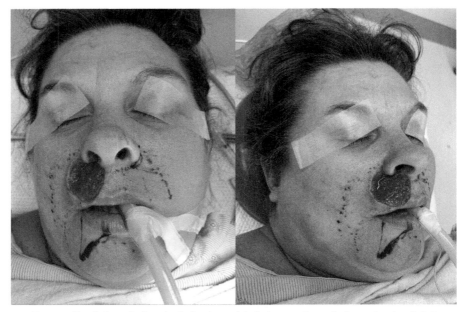

**Fig. 4.** Composite nose/lip defect. Defect includes lateral inferior portion of ala and extends into nasal sill and nasal floor.

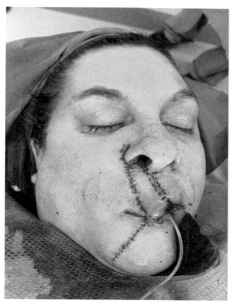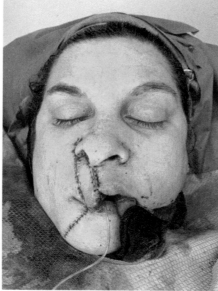

**Fig. 5.** Extended Abbe flap for repair. Lip defect converted to full thickness defect and Abbe flap used to avoid distortion of philtrum from advancement flaps. Medial incision lies on the philtral column. Extended Abbe flap inset to reline floor of nose. Inferior incision designed to lie within mentolabial crease. Secondary nasal reconstruction planned.

thickness skin graft will suffice. In fact, simply healing by secondary intention may sometimes yield the best result. This "laissez-faire" approach is well described, with final esthetic results thought to be equal or perhaps superior to skin grafting in select cases.[9]

More extensive defects may also involve the lower eyelid as part of the medial canthal resection. Additional considerations should be taken into account in these situations. Resection of the lower lacrimal duct may result in persistent epiphora after reconstruction. If partially resected, the surgeon may elect to marsupialize the opening and stent the remaining portion. For cases in which this is not possible, a delayed dacryocysto-rhinostomy is a well-established option for managing epiphora.[10]

Options for lower lid reconstruction depend on whether the defect involves only the anterior lamella, or is a full thickness defect. For composite nasal defects, the cervicofacial flap is often an ideal flap for resurfacing the anterior lamella. Frequently, these large composite defects also involve the medial cheek. As such, a cervicofacial flap can serve to resurface both the eyelid and cheek components (**Figs. 6–8**). A full thickness skin graft is also an option for defects only involving the anterior lamella.

Full thickness defects will require reconstruction of both the anterior and posterior lamella. If a medial anchoring point exists, a Tenzel semicircular flap can mobilize the remaining lateral full thickness eyelid to reconstruct the medial lid. Cervicofacial flaps in conjunction with free tarsoconjunctival grafts for the posterior lamellar reconstruction are also an option. Near total eyelid defects may require staged lid-sharing procedures such as the Hughes tarsoconjunctival flap. Regardless of the method of reconstruction, a key point is the use of any free grafts must be supported by vascularized tissue. If free tarsoconjunctival grafts are to be used for posterior lamella reconstruction, the anterior lamellar reconstruction must be a vascularized flap. The reverse is true if skin grafting is to be used for the anterior lamella; the posterior lamellar reconstruction must be a vascularized flap.[10,11]

## Addressing the Nasal Component

Frequently, the nasal component of composite defects is quite extensive, and a forehead flap will often be the workhorse flap of the nasal reconstruction. Melolabial flaps may be used for nasal defects isolated to the ala or columella but this flap's availability depends on the extent of tissue loss of the ipsilateral cheek.[3,4,8] Thus, the only interpolated option may in fact be the forehead flap. As mentioned already, the key to a successful composite reconstruction is separately reconstructing each of the facial subunits. The approach to complicated defects is often made clearer when creating a separate plan for each involved facial subunit. Once

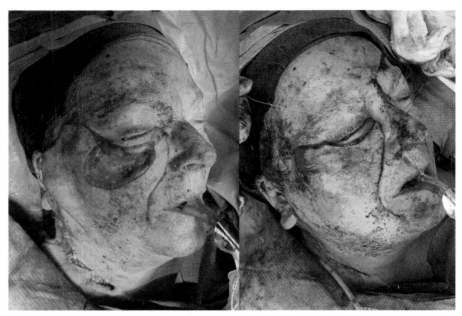

**Fig. 6.** Composite cheek/partial lower lid defect after resection of Merkel cell carcinoma. Cervicofacial flap designed for repair of both subsites. Defect enlarged medially to allow for inset at nasolabial/melolabial crease (*right*). Suture seen securing flap to periosteum of lateral orbital wall.

the midface platform is reestablished, the nasal defect can be addressed using the well-known principles of nasal reconstruction. However, even more so than in an isolated nasal repair, the importance of inner lining and supporting grafts cannot be overstated due to the additional contractile forces of adjacent healing tissues.

### Inner Lining

Inner lining can be addressed in a variety of ways. If the septum is intact, ipsilateral and contralateral septal mucosal hinge flaps can be used to line a hemirhinectomy defect.[4,12] The ipsilateral hinge flap is most useful for more caudally based defects but is not of sufficient surface area to line a larger

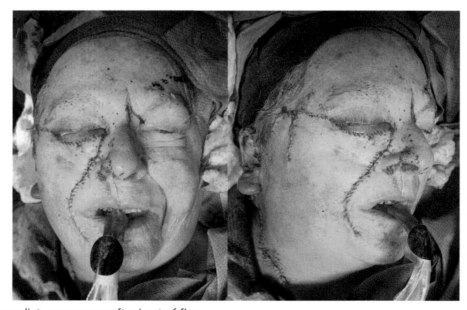

**Fig. 7.** Immediate appearance after inset of flap.

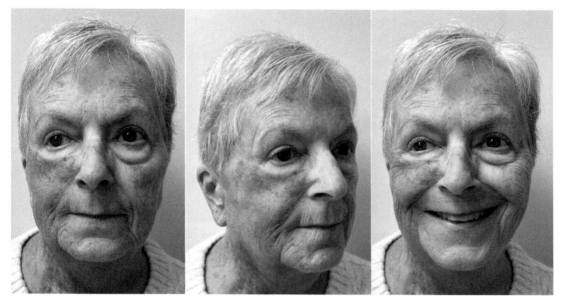

**Fig. 8.** Postoperative results after 6 months; patient also received postoperative radiation.

defect. In such cases, an ipsilateral flap can provide caudal lining while the contralateral flap can reline the nasal midvault. However, large composite defects may include resection of the nasal septum and leave total or near-total nasal defects, leaving the surgeon with a need for different options. A variety of methods have been described in such scenarios. Bilateral forehead flaps can be used, one for inner lining, and one for skin coverage of the nasal defect. Free tissue transfer for inner lining is also a well-established option.

It is the first author's preference not to use bilateral septal mucosal flaps for inner lining if the septum is intact, as doing so necessitates leaving a large septal perforation. Our preference in these situations is the use of laminated or prelaminated forehead flaps, in which the deep surface of the forehead flap is covered with a skin graft. This has multiple advantages. First, it does not require the creation of a large septal perforation if the septum is intact. Second, it remains an outpatient procedure without the need to monitor free tissue transfer. Third, it avoids the need for 2 paramedian forehead flaps with extensive forehead scars. Additionally, although it adds a step to the nasal reconstruction, the flap can often be prelaminated while reconstructing the surrounding tissues at the first stage of reconstruction, with minimal time lost.

The laminated or prelaminated forehead flap is an extension of the 3-stage forehead flap described by Menick.[13] The 3-stage technique is routinely used in our practice for larger nasal defects. The second stage involves completely elevating the paramedian forehead flap while still

leaving it attached to its pedicle. This leaves behind the revascularized inner lining (if the flap was laminated or prelaminated) and soft tissues and allows for excellent and extensive contouring of the nasal tissues with concurrent placement of cartilage or bony supporting grafts (**Fig. 9**). The flap is replaced over the contoured nose and the pedicle divided 3 to 4 weeks later at a third stage.

## Support Grafts

Autologous tissues are preferred whenever possible, although cadaveric rib can be considered. Septal cartilage, if present, is the obvious choice for the creation of nonanatomic sidewall grafts, or in aiding to reconstruct an L-strut. Auricular conchal cartilage grafts are an excellent contour for the reconstruction of the lower lateral cartilage. This can be harvested via an anterior approach with an incision just inside the rim of the conchal bowl, or via a postauricular approach to better hide the incision. The contralateral conchal cartilage is often the best match for the reconstruction of the lateral crus.[3,4]

More extensive dorsal defects or complete loss of the L-strut will require more robust grafts for reconstruction. A cantilevered calvarial bone graft and the central core of rib cartilage sutured to form an L-strut are often the methods of choice.[4,14] The disadvantage of the calvarial bone graft is the need for a coronal approach to access the parietal bone. Patient should be counseled about the low but real risks of dural tears or cerebrospinal fluid leaks. Harvesting rib cartilage has its own set of

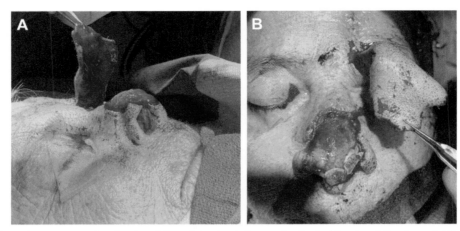

**Fig. 9.** Three-stage paramedian forehead flap. A laminated or prelaminated forehead flap is useful for the nasal component of large nasal defects. Second stage is demonstrated here. Flap is completely elevated in a thin subcutaneous plane but left attached at its pedicle. The underlying soft tissues are visualized. (*A*) The soft tissues can be extensively sculpted and cartilage grafts added at this second stage. (*B*) The paramedian flap is then reinset and divided 3-4 weeks later.

complications including pneumothorax, pleural tears, and injury to the lung. Such complications are readily avoided with a careful harvest but a thorough discussion with the patient before surgery is essential.

## EXTENSIVE TISSUE LOSS

Despite all the local techniques available to the experienced reconstructive surgeon, at times, the extent of tissue resection in large composite resections will leave a volume deficit that simply cannot be overcome with local reconstruction alone. It is these situations in which free flap reconstruction must be considered. The choice of flap depends on the type of tissue needed. If the primary need is for nasal lining, thin pliable tissue will be needed. For larger volume composite defects, a stable midface platform will be needed before nasal reconstruction and bulkier free flaps should be considered. Radial forearm flaps and adipofascial ALT flaps have been described for the reconstruction of nasal inner lining in total nasal defects.[15–17] The additional bulk of soft tissue flaps such as a latissimus or a fasciocutaneous ALT can be excellent options to restore more extensive loss of midface volume (**Figs. 10** and **11**).[18] Extensive maxillary bony defects may require the use of osteocutaneous flaps such as fibula or scapula free flaps to establish a stable midface platform and achieve separation of the oral and nasal cavities.

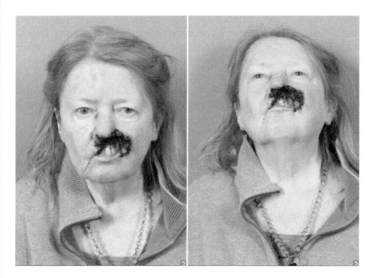

**Fig. 10.** Large basal cell carcinoma eroding nearly the entire upper lip, with involvement of cheek, left commissure, and nasal columella and left ala.

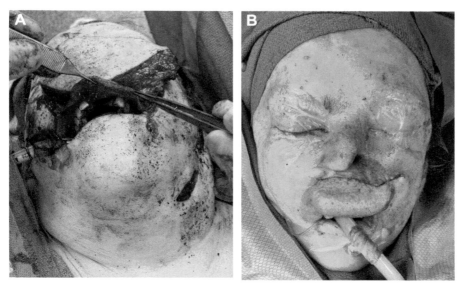

**Fig. 11.** Intraoperative photos patient from **Fig. 10.** Resection defect included entire upper lip, premaxillary tissues, portion of left cheek, left commissure, columella, left ala. Due to volume of tissue loss, local reconstruction, especially for the upper lip, was not feasible. Patient's forearm tissue was extremely thin and not sufficient to reestablish bulk for nasal base; fasciocutaneous ALT was used for initial reconstruction. Fascia was used to restore the vestibule, whereas skin and soft tissue of flap were used to restore midface volume and for lip reconstruction. (A) Patient after first stage of debulking; nasal reconstruction planned at subsequent stages. (B) Despite necessity for free tissue transfer, color and texture match are poor.

Composite defects involving a total or near total upper lip defect may also be strongly considered for free tissue transfer. For the lip, near total upper lip reconstruction is technically possible with Karapandzic flaps or Bernard Burrow flaps. However, Karapandzic flaps can result in severe microstomia. Additionally, large defects may include lip and cheek tissues, precluding the use of cheek-recruiting flaps such as the Bernard Burrow flaps. Thus, at times, the only feasible option may be free tissue transfer.

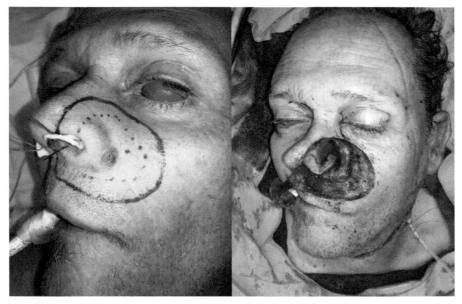

**Fig. 12.** Basal cell carcinoma, resulting in a large composite defect of nose, white upper lip, and medial cheek tissues. Staged reconstruction of the cheek and lip was planned.

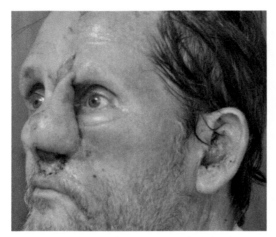

**Fig. 13.** Same patient from **Fig. 12**, after cheek and lip reconstruction, with subsequent inset of paramedian forehead flap.

In cases requiring free tissue transfer, if it is possible to restore the deeper tissue volume with the free flap and resurface with adjacent tissues, the overall results will esthetically be superior. This concept is similar to using the previously discussed SMAS flap for volume and a separate cervicofacial flap for skin covering. In more extensive defects, the free flap tissue can "fill the hole" to restore bulk and volume, while secondary staged local flaps, such as large cervicofacial flaps, can resurface the skin. As always, replacing "like with like" is the goal. A face resurfaced with distant skin will always be a poorer color and texture match for reconstruction (see **Fig. 11**).[18]

## REPRESENTATIVE CASE

A 45-year-old man with biopsy confirmed basal cell carcinoma underwent wide local excision with negative margins (**Fig. 12**). Resection resulted in a large composite defect involving all 3 layers of the nose, multiple nasal subunits, and multiple facial units including the left cheek and white lip (see **Fig. 12**). Further analysis of the defect revealed the following.

1. Left medial cheek defect including loss of skin and soft tissue depth down to the medial maxilla.
2. Half of the height of the left superior white lip skin including the superior left philtrum column.
3. Total thickness loss of left ala, left soft tissue triangle, left half of columella, left nasal sidewall, and a portion of the lobule and dorsum.
4. Loss of left floor of nose mucosa, caudal septal mucosa.

To approach this patient, the involved facial units were identified and separately reconstruction. A large rolled SMAS flap was advanced medially and tacked to bone anchored sutures through the maxilla to address the volume loss of the medial cheek. For the cutaneous component, a large

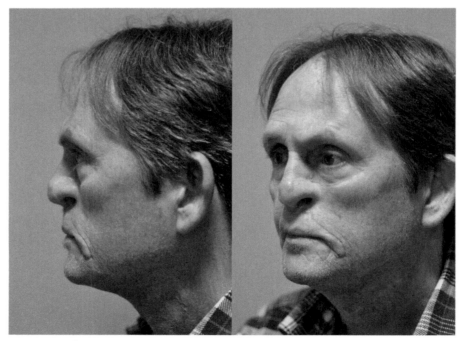

**Fig. 14.** Same patient after additional nasal contouring procedures; patient declined further reconstruction at this stage.

cheek advancement flap with incisions in the eye-cheek esthetic unit border and nasolabial regions was used to complete the cheek repair. The lip defect was addressed with full thickness skin grafts harvested from the left supraclavicular region. The nasal reconstruction was staged after first addressing the cheek and lip defects.

The approach to the complex nasal defect required multiple techniques. A left-sided posteriorly based septomucosal flap was raised and draped along the floor of nose to repair this defect. Septal cartilage was harvested leaving a 1-cm caudal and dorsal strut. A posteriorly pedicled septomucosal flap from the right side was tunneled through the defect of the septal perforation to provide inner lining to the midvault on the left side. The harvested septal cartilage provided structure to the midvault. Composite ear cartilage grafting (anterior conchal bowl skin and cartilage) was used to reconstruct the nasal ala and soft tissue triangle. Laterally, the composite graft was anchored to the bone of the maxilla. The columella was reconstructed with a composite ear graft and a full thickness skin graft. The nasal skin was resurfaced with a paramedian forehead flap (**Fig. 13**).

After division of forehead flap and several contouring operations, the patient wished to discontinue further surgical treatment (**Fig. 14**). Note that despite the apparent large initial defect, free tissue transfer was not necessary for reconstruction, and local options resulted in a better color match and skin texture for the patient.

## SUMMARY

Composite nasal defects complicate what is often already a very challenging nasal reconstruction. Breaking down the defect in terms of the involved facial subunits can help to simplify these complex reconstructions. Surgeons should focus on developing a separate plan for each involved unit and avoid the temptation to use a large flap simply to just "fill the hole." Deeper defects should be staged, and a stable midfacial platform should be established before the nasal portion of the surgery. Although every attempt should be made to use local flaps, the extent of large composite defects will still occasionally require the use of free tissue transfer. In such situations, the distal tissue should be used to restore volume and bulk, and the defect should be resurfaced with adjacent tissues if feasible.

## CLINICS CARE POINTS

- Planning for composite nasal defects should delineate the involved facial subunits.

- Develop a separate reconstructive plan for each involved facial unit; avoid simply "filling the hole."
- Establish a stable midface platform before proceeding with nasal reconstruction.
- Consider staging nasal reconstruction after the cheek and lip are first addressed.
- Free tissue transfer should be used for volume replacement and resurfaced with local flaps when feasible.

## DISCLOSURE

The authors have no commercial or financial interests to disclose.

## REFERENCES

1. Burget GC, Menick FJ. The subunit principle in nasal reconstruction. Plast Reconstr Surg 1985;76(2):239–47.
2. Menick FJ. Defects of the nose, lip, and cheek: rebuilding the composite defect. Plast Reconstr Surg 2007;120(4):887–98.
3. Austin GK, Shockley WW. Reconstruction of nasal defects: contemporary approaches. Curr Opin Otolaryngol Head Neck Surg 2016;24(5):453–60.
4. Tollefson TT, Kriet JD. Complex nasal defects: structure and internal lining. Facial Plast Surg Clin North Am 2005;13(2):333–vii.
5. Owusu J, Nesbitt B, Boahene K. Management of complicated nasal defects. Facial Plast Surg 2020;36(2):158–65.
6. Pletcher SD, Kim DW. Current concepts in cheek reconstruction. Facial Plast Surg Clin North Am 2005;13(2):267, vi.
7. Chu MW, Dobratz EJ. Reconstruction of the dorsal and sidewall defects. Facial Plast Surg Clin North Am 2011;19(1):13–24.
8. Baker S. Chapter 19. Reconstruction of the lips. In: Baker S, editor. Local flaps in facial reconstruction. 3rd edition. Philadelphia, PA: Saunders/Elsevier; 2014. p. 481–528.
9. Shafi F, Rathore D, Johnson A, et al. Medial canthal defects following tumour excision: To reconstruct or not to reconstruct? Orbit 2017;36(2):64–8.
10. Madge SN, Malhotra R, Thaller VT, et al. A systematic approach to the oculoplastic reconstruction of the eyelid medial canthal region after cancer excision. Int Ophthalmol Clin 2009;49(4):173–94.
11. Mukit M, Anbar F, Dadireddy K, et al. Eyelid reconstruction: an algorithm based on defect location. J Craniofac Surg 2022;33(3):821–6.
12. Joseph AW, Truesdale C, Baker SR. Reconstruction of the nose. Facial Plast Surg Clin North Am 2019;27(1):43–54.

13. Menick FJ. Forehead flap: master techniques in otolaryngology-head and neck surgery. Facial Plast Surg 2014;30(2):131–44.

14. Shipchandler TZ, Chung BJ, Alam DS. Saddle nose deformity reconstruction with a split calvarial bone L-shaped strut. Arch Facial Plast Surg 2008;10(5): 305–11.

15. Revenaugh PC, Haffey TM, Seth R, et al. Antero-lateral thigh adipofascial flap in mucosal reconstruction. JAMA Facial Plast Surg 2014;16(6): 395–9.

16. Seth R, Revenaugh PC, Scharpf J, et al. Free antero-lateral thigh fascia lata flap for complex nasal lining defects. JAMA Facial Plast Surg 2013;15(1):21–8.

17. Winslow CP, Cook TA, Burke A, et al. Total nasal reconstruction: utility of the free radial forearm fascial flap. Arch Facial Plast Surg 2003;5(2):159–63.

18. Burget GC, Walton RL. Optimal use of microvascular free flaps, cartilage grafts, and a paramedian forehead flap for aesthetic reconstruction of the nose and adjacent facial units. Plast Reconstr Surg 2007;120(5):1171–207.

# Prevention and Management of Complications in Nasal Reconstruction

Hannah N. Kuhar, MD, Ryan Nesemeier, MD, Leslie R. Kim, MD*

## KEYWORDS

- Nasal reconstruction • Complications • Prevention • Management

## KEY POINTS

- Nasal reconstruction is a complicated process that requires extensive preparation by the surgeon to prevent and manage potential complications that can occur across preoperative, intraoperative, and postoperative settings.
- In the preoperative setting, modifiable and nonmodifiable patient factors should be optimized in order to prevent potential complications.
- Intraoperatively, the surgeon can prevent complications through proper sterile practices and meticulous surgical technique.
- In the postoperative setting, attentive wound care, early identification of need for revision, and the addition of adjuvant therapies allow for the effective mitigation and management of complications.

## INTRODUCTION

Nasal reconstruction is rooted in both form and function of the nose. The nose is the most central and prominent feature of the face that lacks donor tissue with the same composition. Therefore, nasal reconstruction is a practice of camouflaging dissimilar tissues to resemble those of a "normal" nose, rather than rebuilding from what remains. Nasal reconstruction requires adequate attention to each of the nasal anatomic elements of the outer cover (skin and soft tissues), structure (bone, cartilage, and fibrofatty tissue), and lining (mucosa and vestibular skin).[1] Complications encountered from nasal reconstruction are sometimes anticipated preoperatively but may also be encountered both intraoperative and postoperatively. Residual nasal deformities following complex nasal reconstruction are common, and the need for adjuvant conservative treatments or staged additional procedures should be anticipated.[1]

Opportunity exists for the identification and prevention of potential complications in the perioperative period. In the preoperative setting, emphasis should be placed on the identification of and optimization of individual patient risk factors that might affect wound healing. Intraoperatively, the surgeon should focus on techniques that protect against complications. Postoperatively, vigilant wound care and close follow-up may prevent avoidable complications while allowing for early detection and intervention in complications that arise.

## DISCUSSION

### Prevention of Complications in the Preoperative Period

#### Modifiable risk factors

#### Patient nutrition

- Optimizing patient nutrition is important for enhanced wound healing.[2]

Department of Otolaryngology–Head and Neck Surgery, Ohio State University Wexner Medical Center, Ohio State Eye and Ear Institute, 915 Olentangy River Road, Suite 4000, Columbus, OH 43212, USA
* Corresponding author.
E-mail address: Leslie.Kim@osumc.edu

Facial Plast Surg Clin N Am 32 (2024) 303–313
https://doi.org/10.1016/j.fsc.2024.01.009
1064-7406/24/© 2024 Elsevier Inc. All rights reserved.

- Vitamins A, C, and iron are required for collagen synthesis. Zinc is required for epithelialization.[3] Immunonutrition, such as arginine amino acid supplementation, has been associated with increased collagen synthesis and stimulation of lymphocyte and growth hormone production critical to wound healing.[2,3]
- Preoperative carbohydrate loading, such as a carbohydrate drink on the night before and the morning of the procedure, has been associated with reduced insulin resistance, less loss of lean body mass and muscle strength, as well as decreased length of hospitalization.[2]

## Smoking

- Smoking is well known to negatively affect healing, through tissue hypoxia and microvasculature thrombosis. Smoking increases the risk of complications, including infection, wound dehiscence, and skin necrosis secondary to nicotine.[4]
- Nicotine activates the adrenergic nervous system and causes systemic vasoconstriction, potentially lowering tissue oxygenation pressure over 50%.[5] Nicotine increases the risk of skin necrosis secondary to endothelial thickening and damage to small vessels of the skin, as well as vasoconstriction.[6] Carbon monoxide from smoking has a higher affinity for hemoglobin than oxygen, creating high levels of carboxyhemoglobin with less oxygen delivered to tissues.[7]
- Ideally, procedures should be delayed until smoking cessation is confirmed.[8] Among patients undergoing nasal reconstruction with forehead flap, smokers have higher odds of developing flap necrosis.[9] Recommended time of smoking cessation varies in the literature. One recommendation is smoking cessation for 2 months prior and 1 month after surgery.[9] The authors recommend smoking cessation for 3 to 6 weeks prior to and after surgery.
- Nicotine replacement therapy should be considered in cases where smoking cessation is not possible. Clinical experimental studies have demonstrated that smoking cessation with nicotine patch normalizes cutaneous microvascular perfusion.[10,11] When compared to smoking, nicotine replacement therapy did not affect glucose or lactate levels of tissue metabolism.[11] In abstinent smokers receiving either active or placebo nicotine patches, the active patch did not affect angiogenesis, wound contraction, or epidermal regeneration.[12]

## Medications and supplements

- Preoperative screening should be performed to identify any prescription and over-the-counter medications or supplements that may contribute to perioperative bleeding.[7]
- All aspirin-containing products, nonsteroidal anti-inflammatory medicines, Vitamin E, and herbal supplements (such as ginkgo biloba, ginseng, chondroitin-glucosamine, melatonin, turmeric, bilberry, chamomile, fenugreek, milk thistle, and peppermint) should be discontinued at least 1 week prior to surgery.[13,14] Decongestant cold/sinus medications should be avoided preoperatively because they may influence bleeding and blood pressure.[7]
- In cases where a pre-existing medical condition requires continuation of these medications, preoperative clearance by relevant subspecialists should take place.[15]

## Nonmodifiable risk factors
### Skin conditions

- A variety of nonmodifiable patient factors affect wound healing outcomes, such as Fitzpatrick skin type and age.[15] Patients may be stratified according to their individual preoperative risk for complications.[5]
  - Fair-skinned patients develop scars that remain pink for an extended interval, while darker skinned individuals (Fitzpatrick types III–VI) are more likely to form hyperpigmented or keloid scars.
  - History of poor scarring should be elicited in the medical history.
  - Children and young adults are more likely to develop thick, firm scars. Scar revision is often delayed until after puberty.
  - Skin conditions such as psoriasis or atrophic dermatitis present an increased risk of healing complications.[7,8]

### Radiation history

- In cases of irradiated tissues, the surgeon must balance delaying reconstruction with the risk of scar contracture over time.[7] Reconstruction should not delay radiation, which is recommended to begin within 6 weeks after ablative surgery. If it cannot be completed within this timeframe, it is recommended to delay reconstruction until 3 to 6 months after the completion of radiation.[16] Perioperative hyperbaric oxygen therapy (HBO) may be considered in these cases pending clearance from the oncologic team and patient risk factors (emphysema, and so forth).[17]

## Medical comorbidities

- Knowledge of patient medical history is critical for preoperative optimization of healing. Communication with primary or specialist physicians managing the patient's pre-existing medical conditions is important to prevent complications.[7]
- Steroid use for chronic disease, use of anti-metabolites for cancer, coagulation disorders, thyroid disease, or history of prior surgery at or adjacent to defect present an increased risk of wound healing complications.[7,8]
- Patients with diabetes are at an increased risk of perioperative infection. A HgbA1c level less than 7% has been associated with decreased perioperative infectious complications.[18] Serum glucose levels should be monitored closely in the perioperative period.[7]
- Immunocompromised patients on immuno-suppressive therapy may have delayed wound healing and require "stress dose" steroids in the perioperative period.[15]
- Individuals with hyperelastic joints and more dermal elastin will be more likely to form widened scars.[5,15]
- If there is any concern for easy bruising or bleeding, consider hematology evaluation for the possibility of an underlying hematologic disorder.[7]

## Psychosocial screening

- Medical history taking should also include psychosocial screening, in order to understand the patient's mindset, expectations, and social support ahead of surgery.[5]
- A thorough consent process should take place preoperatively. Consent should include discussion about surgical planning, including the potential for staged or additional procedures, in order to help define patient expectations.

## Prevention of Complications in the Intraoperative Period

### Sterile technique

- Intraoperative sterile technique is important to avoid infection. Skin preparation with anti-septic solution, sterile technique, and sterile surgical attire are critical.[7]

### Antibiotic use

- Perioperative antibiotic prophylaxis is associated with decreased wound infection in clean-contaminated wounds.[7]
- Antibiotics should be utilized when mucosal surfaces are incised, cartilage grafting is performed and when ear cartilage is used to avoid perichondritis.[7,15]
- Antibiotics are also recommended when patients have pre-existing medical conditions that predispose to infection or in open wounds older than 3 days.[7]
- The authors frequently employ intraoperative weight-based cefazolin, followed by a week-long course of trimethoprim-sulfamethoxazole or amoxicillin-clavulanic acid twice daily in cases of nasal reconstruction. When cartilage grafting is used, consider coverage with anti-pseudomonal antibiotics such as fluoroquino-lones, which have been successful in treating auricular perichondritis and may be periopera-tively implemented as prophylactic antibiotics during reconstructive procedures involving exposed cartilage.[19] It is important to take note of medication allergies/sensitivities when prescribing antibiotics.

### Flap design

- Intraoperatively, meticulous flap design is necessary to prevent unfavorable scarring. Multiple factors, including inappropriate placement of incisions, poorly designed local flaps, and wound location and size, may contribute to unfavorable scarring.[15]
- When possible, the surgeon should mimic the contralateral structures when designing flaps, taking care to respect the nasal subunits and use them as guides for scars. Suture foil or Telfa nonadherent dressing can be used to create templates.
- Surgical techniques that affect scar development include failure to properly approximate and evert wound edges, failure to obtain tension-free wound closure, and removal of cutaneous sutures in an untimely manner.[15]
- Trap-door deformity may occur from edema and poor lymphatic drainage in flaps with curvilinear borders, such as bilobed flaps. Patients with thick nasal skin and sebaceous gland hypertrophy are at highest risk. Superi-orly based flaps are at higher risk of trap-door deformity due to the inferior orientation of facial lymphatic drainage. Trap-door defor-mity is avoided by wide undermining and proper flap design. Squaring of edges, rather than rounding, has been shown to reduce the development of trap-door deformities.[20]

### Multilayer reconstruction

- The nasal framework includes 9 esthetic sub-units. Total nasal subunit reconstruction should take place when a defect involves

50% or more of a subunit. Reconstruction requires attention to the 3 lamellae of the nose, which are lining, support, and coverage.[1] Awareness of nasal subunit-specific challenges is necessary for the prevention and management of complications.

- Failure to reconstruct all layers results in unfavorable scarring. In particular, deficient lining reconstruction is a major cause of delayed poor healing because it results in delayed contracture of the overlying cover layer.
- Bosuk and colleagues (2021) discuss potential complications for nasal cover reconstruction of each subunit (**Table 1**).

### Flap design-specific considerations for prevention of complications
#### Timing of surgery
- Timing of facial reconstruction is important. For large defects, consider staging cheek and lip reconstruction first, in order to build a stable base for nasal reconstruction.[8]

#### Facial esthetic regions and units
- Facial esthetic regions and units should be respected when designing cutaneous flaps to avoid unfavorable scars.[7] Cutaneous defects extending from the nose to the medial cheek or upper lip should be repaired with separate flaps for each esthetic region to better camouflage scars in boundary lines.

#### Facial feature distortion
- Over time, scar contracture can affect mobile facial structures of eyelids, lips, and nasal alae.[7] It is important to anticipate the potential for long-term facial feature distortion. Flaps should be secured to the periosteum of the nasal bones or maxilla to reduce wound closure tension.

#### Incision placement
- Placement of incisions within subunit borders helps to camouflage reconstructive techniques, whereas those that cross tend to be more noticeable and less desirable.
- Closure should be performed parallel to or within relaxed skin tension lines where possible.[15]

#### Defect preparation
- Recipient bed preparation is critical for nutrient diffusion, neoangiogenesis, and graft uptake.[7]
- Wound edges should be freshened and the inward beveled edges that result from Mohs excision corrected to facilitate uniform thickness and skin eversion.
- Wound thickness should guide selection of the graft site. Wound levels are typically taken down through the superficial musculoaponeurotic system layer to facilitate full-thickness repair for improved esthetic outcomes.
- Intraoperatively, crushed, charred, or excessively thinned tissue should be discarded.[7]

#### Protecting surrounding structures
- Injury to surrounding structures should be avoided at all costs. Injury to the underlying nasal cartilage can lead to deformities such as alar retraction, nasal valve collapse, saddle nose deformity, and tip asymmetries. Tension around the eye can lead to lagophthalmos, lacrimal duct obstruction, visual field obstruction, and vision loss.[7,15]

#### Nonanatomic grafting
- Nasal flaps should be designed large enough to avoid alar retraction. Alar rim defects should use cartilage grafting to resist external nasal valve compromise. Frequently, nonanatomic grafting is used in the nasal alar region to resist collapse under the weight of the flap and because the dense fibrofatty tissue present within the alar is not found in other donor tissues.[21]
- Cartilage grafts are immobilized with sutures and tight pockets within surrounding tissues to facilitate incorporation and prevent distortion.[16]

#### Ischemia
- Reconstruction technique should ensure perfusion of the flap tissue. Local and regional flaps can have either random or axial perfusion patterns, which affects the depth of dissection.[7]
- Increasing the width of a flap may increase the number of subdermal plexus vessels, but this does not increase perfusion pressure to the distal portion of the flap. Properly designed templates should be used to estimate the native tissues for appropriate flap size. Axial pattern flaps rely on a specific artery within the flap tissue and require a thicker flap with deeper subcutaneous vessels, parallel to the linear axis of the flap. Doppler of contributing vessels or standard measurements may be implemented during flap planning.
- Flap closure wounds are at an increased risk of tissue ischemia than wounds that are primarily closed. Flap dissection causes the release of catecholamines from sympathetic

**Table 1**
**Reconstruction options by nasal site and complication considerations**

| Nasal Site | Reconstruction Options | Complication Considerations |
|---|---|---|
| Nasal dorsum | Upper third and middle third defects<br>• Random dorsal nasal sliding flaps, glabellar flaps, and axial flaps from the inferior trochlear and external ethmoidal arteries | • Distortion of the natural dorsal esthetic lines, medial brow position, and nasolabial tip angulation<br>• Optimal nasal dorsum reconstruction involves taking tissue from outside the nasal esthetic subunits, such as the axial forehead flap, to avoid distortion of the nasal appearance and architecture<br>• Tension-free closure is difficult with these flaps |
| | Lower third defects<br>• Locoregional flaps and bilobed flaps | • Nasal distortion<br>• In the case of bilobed flaps, cicatricial depression between the 2 flaps may develop, as well as pin-cushioning during scar healing |
| Nasal sidewall | Upper nasal sidewall and medial canthal defects<br>• Full-thickness skin grafting | • Color mismatch |
| | Middle and distal sidewall defects<br>• Nasolabial flaps or bilobed flaps<br>• Two-stage inferior facial artery–based nasolabial flap<br>• V-Y nasolabial flap<br>• Lateral nasal artery flap (Rybka type)<br>• Island forehead flap | • Pin-cushioning and standing cutaneous defects at the donor sites<br>• When tissue is borrowed from outside of the nose, there is lower chance of nasal distortion |
| Nasal tip | • Forehead flap reconstruction is typically necessary unless the defect is very small, to resurface the entire esthetic unit<br>• Nasal sidewall flaps or dorsal tissue flaps will distort the nose and should be avoided | • Circular flap design that distorts the nasal tip unit shape with scar contracture and causes a pin-cushion deformity |
| Nasal alae | • Bilobed flaps are frequently implemented<br>• Two-stage inferior facial artery–based nasolabial flap and lateral nasal artery island flaps for small defects of 7 mm or less<br>• Defects >50% of the subunit or full-thickness defects require staged forehead flaps for coverage ± cartilage grafting. Specific attention must be placed to resurfacing the entire alar unit, not just the defect, with emphasis on a curved alar rim that inserts into the columella | • Pin-cushioning and scar contracture<br>• Distortion of the natural alar crease<br>• Complications from incomplete alar reconstruction. Flap revision with thinning and sculpting in subsequent procedures is often necessary |
| Soft triangle | • Specific considerations for the soft triangle include that it is the same in color as the nasal tip subunit<br>• Mucosa-based total alar V-Y advancement flaps can be implemented to maintain mucosal perfusion to the soft tissue, however may distort the alar sill appearance | • Esthetically sensitive to color mismatch. For example, auricular composite grafts can frequently case color mismatch and alar distortion |

*Data from* Bosuk et al (2021).[1]

nerves, thromboxane A from platelet micro-thrombi, and oxygen free radicals, which together promote ischemia. Anticipation of which portion of a specific flap is at highest risk for ischemia is important. Rotation or advancement flaps have the greatest wound closure tension at the distal closure site, whereas transposition flaps have greater wound closure tension at the donor site.

**Intraoperative measures to promote flap survival**
- Intraoperatively, flap vascularity is promoted by avoiding excessive tissue thinning, electro-cautery, crush injury with surgical instruments, and wound closure tension. Superficial dissection or improper flap design may compromise flap vascularity.[7] Similarly, sutures for inset should largely be kept in the cutaneous plane because subcutaneous sutures may affect the subdermal plexus needed for survival and integration. Sutures should be placed in a simple fashion and the flap frequently assessed for appropriate color. If the flap appears pale after placement of sutures, remove them as necessary.
- Local anesthetic with vasoconstrictor agents should be used judiciously due to the potential for flap ischemia and distortion of tissue planes.
- Flaps should be frequently reassessed during elevation to ensure perfusion at the distal aspect. If at any point there seems to be compromise, it is best to delay the flap by partially reinsetting into the donor site.

**Hemostasis**
- Intraoperative hemostasis is necessary for visualization and hematoma prevention.
- Collection of blood beneath the flap may compromise vascularity.[7]

**Tension-free wound closure**
- Tension-free wound closure is critical for the prevention of scar formation. Incisions near mobile structures are at greatest risk for hypertrophic and apparent scarring. Thick-skinned areas, such as the caudal nose, are most likely to produce noticeable scars.[15]

### Flap-specific technical refinements for prevention of complications
#### Paramedian forehead flap
- Paramedian forehead flaps (PMFF) should be dissected down to the subgaleal plane, allowing for easier primary donor site closure and healing by secondary intent.
- Flaps should be thinned either at the first or second stage. At the first stage, thinning can

take place down to the level of the subdermal vascular plexus, maintaining 2 to 3 mm of subcutaneous adipose tissue.[22] If there is any question of flap compromise, thinning should be delayed.
- PMFF complication rates range from 1% to 31% and include flap congestion, dehiscence, nasal obstruction, and surgical site infections.[5] Cartilage grafting is associated with an increased risk of complications, likely due to increased complexity of the reconstruction and the potential for cartilage warping over time.[5]
- Flap necrosis is typically due to excessive tension, failure to identify past injury to its pedicle or scar in the region of the flap, or overaggressive flap thinning.
- When flap compromise is suspected, early debridement and possible coverage with a second flap may be preferred to healing by secondary intention.[6,8]
- Infection most often occurs from failure of aseptic technique or lining necrosis, which may require revision and/or skin grafting with delayed reconstruction of primary support. In chronic infections, preference is for limited flap re-elevation and cartilage debridement, with secondary support reconstruction later.[8] Nitropaste is frequently applied proactively when there is any concern for vascular flap compromise.[23]
- It is imperative when performing PMFFs to accurately measure the length of the pedicle. This can be done by using a surgical sponge placed at the orbital bone at the area of the supratrochlear artery and stretching it to the most distal aspect of the defect. There should be enough redundancy of the sponge to allow for a lack of tension on the flap. The sponge can then be rotated medially (as the flap would) onto the forehead to estimate the length necessary for the flap. This can be repeated 3 times, each time using a new section or piece of the sponge to ensure the same length each time. If additional flap length is necessary to reduce tension when elevating, this can be taken down below the orbital bone, taking care to protect the artery, which typically exits from the orbit. This is usually accomplished by elevating in the subperiosteal plane, which may begin approximately 10 mm from the orbit.
- If there is distal flap compromise, an intermediate procedure can be performed in which the forehead flap is raised and further advanced distally by making additional incisions below the brow as described above.

## Lateral nasal artery flap

- The lateral nasal artery flap is based on the watershed junction of the angular and facial arteries, and it can be designed with either a superiorly or inferiorly based pedicle mobilized up to 1.5 cm.[1]
- Flap dissection must preserve venous outflow and have a wider base to include the nutrient artery. The flap should descend to the cheek laterally within the alar groove to avoid nasal alar retraction. Flaps should be thinned to match normal nasal thickness.

## Melolabial flap

- Melolabial flaps are used as one-stage superiorly based angular artery flaps or 2-stage inferiorly based facial artery flaps.[8]
- The 1-stage flap risks standing cutaneous deformity (dog ear) and obscures normal esthetic lines of the nose, resulting in potential pin-cushioning of the flap from a superiorly based pedicle and round-tip design. Pin-cushioning occurs from poor venous drainage and swelling and circumferential scar contracture.[1] A second stage procedure is often required.
- Inferiorly based 2-stage flaps for nasal alar defects provide better venous drainage and improved natural nasal esthetic line definition.
- Melolabial crease scarring and possible lip position distortion are possible.

## Bilobed flap

- Complications include pin-cushioning and depression between the first and second flaps.[1]
- Complications are prevented with wider and inferiorly based pedicle to reduce swelling. Conversion of round defects into square defects also help to combat the "cicatricial tourniquet" that occurs as the scars heal.[1] Prophylactic massage starting 2 weeks postoperatively may aid with swelling. Corticosteroid injection of the flap may also be done, with delayed thinning procedures as the last resort.[1]

## Prevention of Complications in the Postoperative Period

Several factors affect wound healing following nasal reconstruction. Wounds heal through 3 stages following initial coagulation, including an inflammatory phase with re-epithelialization, a fibroblastic phase and a maturation phase with collagen deposition. Wound healing is influenced by the type of injury, location, and local cellular and humoral responses.[15]

Maintenance of a moist local wound environment immediately after reconstruction is necessary for healing. Occlusive or semiocclusive dressings positioned over wounds promote re-epithelialization by secondary intention. Skin grafts and composite grafts may require bolster dressings to prevent shearing and graft loss. Exposed tissue of interpolated flap pedicles should be covered.[24]

Silicone scar sheeting is thought to improve scar healing through hydration effects. The moist wound environment allows for increased oxygen tension in the skin, decreased angiogenesis, local tissue hypoxia, reduction in mast cell concentration, and subsequent decreased histamine production that reduces the size and thickness of scars. Silicone oil is also thought to directly create a negative static electric field that reduces the vascularity of the scar.[25]

In nasal reconstruction, wound healing is a complex process because surgeons are frequently rebuilding multiple layers of the nasal framework and utilizing external tissue for reconstruction. There is a spectrum of complications that can occur postoperatively requiring various levels of response. Judicious early and regular postoperative follow-up is needed in order to recognize and address wound healing complications in a timely fashion.[7,15]

### Postoperative hypothermia

- Specifically in the case of composite grafts, postoperative hypothermia reduces metabolic demands of the graft tissue and enhances graft survival.[26] Cooling takes place through direct application of cold compresses or ice to the surgical site, which creates a bacteriostatic environment to promote healing and decrease metabolic demands of reconstructed tissue. Several protocols have been described, including a 72-hour cooling regimen ahead of neovascularization during postoperative days 3 to 5.[26]

### Perioperative oral steroids

- Perioperative steroids may decrease the metabolic demands of grafted tissue through inhibition of phospholipase and inflammatory mediators, stabilization of cell membranes, stimulation of gluconeogenesis, and reduction of lactic acid levels.[26] Steroid regimens, ranging from a 3-day course of methylprednisolone to a 7-day prednisone taper (eg, 60 mg to 5 mg, taper by 10 mg daily) have been described.[26] Steroids have not been shown to be effective for graft salvage once necrosis is apparent.[26]

### Other pharmacologic agents

- Heparin, topical nitroglycerin, allopurinol, melatonin, nonsteroidal anti-inflammatory drugs (eg, ibuprofen and indomethacin), and oxygen-free radical scavengers (eg, chlorpromazine, dimethylsulfoxide, and superoxide dismutase) have been proposed to improve graft survival. The mechanism of enhanced survival is thought to be the antithrombotic, vasodilatory, and/or anti-inflammatory properties of the agents.[26] Dimethylsulfoxide, chlorpromazine, and indomethacin preoperatively, with indomethacin for 3 days postoperatively, have also been shown to promote composite graft tissue survival.[27]

### Leeches

- Leeches may be used for flap venous congestion in the immediate postoperative period for any concern of potential necrosis and can last from 4 to 10 days.[28,29] By actively extracting blood, leeches increase perfusion within congested tissue. Additionally, leech secretions include the anticoagulant hirudin, histamine-like vasodilators, enzymes (ie, collagenase, apyrase, and hyaluronidase), and calin platelet aggregation inhibitor.[30] Local injection of bivalirudin, a recombinant hirudin derivative, has also been used as a method of "pharmacologic leeching," with improved flap survival seen in cases of venous congestion.[31]
- Oral ciprofloxacin or trimethoprim-sulfamethoxazole prophylaxis is necessary to prevent infection with *Aeromonas hydrophila*.

### Hyperbaric oxygen

- Hyperbaric oxygen (HBO) may enhance the survival of flaps and grafts, particularly composite grafts, grafts that are more tenuous due to size (eg, >1 cm), or compromised wound beds.[26] HBO delivers 100% oxygen inspiration at pressures greater than 1 atm, maximizing oxygen diffusion through tissues and wound healing capacity. HBO has been found to increase fluid diffusion distance by up to 5-fold and is used for chronic wounds, osteomyelitis, and postradiation soft tissue complications.[26,32]

### Adjuvant regenerative medicine approaches
### Platelet-rich plasma

- Platelet-rich plasma (PRP) maintains a high concentration of functional bioactive molecules (transforming growth factor [TGF]-β1, TGF-β2, epidermal growth factor, fibroblast growth factor, platelet-derived growth factor, vascular endothelial growth factor, and interleukin-1) thought to promote graft survival. To date, the majority of studies rely on animal data.[26] In humans, PRP application to split thickness skin grafts has been demonstrated to enhance graft uptake.[33] Additionally, application of PRP has a beneficial effect in cases of bone grafting, fat grafting, and overall wound healing in humans.[34,35]

### Adipose-derived stem cells

- Adipose-derived stem cells (ADSCs) have been used for enhanced wound healing and as a cartilage-substitute for structural support in nasal reconstruction.[36,37] ADSCs secrete cytokines and growth factors that prevent mucosal injury. The cells mimic histologic, functional, and mechanical qualities of native nasal septal cartilage by attaching cells to a scaffold and allowing them to expand and secrete matrix components. Protocols to develop consistent ADSC tissue engineering for nasal reconstruction are under investigation.[36]

## Management of Early Complications in the Postoperative Period

### Hematomas

- Hematomas compromise local flap vascularity by inducing vasospasm, stretching the subdermal plexus, or separating the flap from the surface of the recipient site. Hematomas may also contain iron compounds that promote free radical production, flap necrosis, and predispose to infection.

### Infection

- Facial tissues have abundant vascularity and overall low rates of infection.
- Infection occurs in the setting of inflammatory edema. Release of toxic substances and free radicals from inflammatory mediators lead to decreased collagen production and early degradation of suture materials and wound dehiscence.
- Close monitoring is necessary for early detection of wound infections. Signs of infection include excess pain or erythema at the surgical site as well as foul odor when necrotic tissue exists.
- Antibiotic ointments containing polymyxin or bacitracin should not be applied for longer than 4 to 5 days because there is the risk of

skin reaction that may be confused for infection.

- Gram staining and culture should be performed. Appropriate broad-spectrum antibiotics should be started. Wounds should be drained, irrigated, and/or debrided as indicated.

### Wound dehiscence

- Wound separation may occur due to excessive dynamic motion/trauma, infection, hematoma, or skin necrosis. Repair with suture is reserved only for uncomplicated, clean wounds within 24 hours. Any dehiscence older than 24 hours should heal by secondary intention.

## Management of Late Complications in the Postoperative Period

### Abnormal scarring

- Incisions closed with excessive wound closure tension will yield hypopigmented and hypertrophied scars.
- Thick skin incisions with sebaceous gland hypertrophy will yield depressed or widened scars.
- Hyperpigmentation occurs in patients with excessive sun exposure postoperatively.
- Scar revision in children should be delayed due to their increased scar erythema and hypertrophy.
- Scar tissue volume can be reduced with intralesional injection of triamcinolone acetonide (Kenalog(R) - Bristol-Myers Squibb [New Brunswick, NJ]). Steroid injections reduce fibrosis and excessive formation of scar tissue by decreasing fibroblast activity, reducing neovascularization, and disrupting fibrosis through inhibition of extracellular matrix protein gene expression. Injections are performed subdermally and as a series. Various types and concentrations have been reported. Commonly, triamcinolone acetonide at 10 mg/mL is implemented.[24] Scar excision with perioperative intralesional injections may be performed if the scar is responsive. Risks of steroid injections include skin atrophy, hypopigmentation, and telangiectasia.
- Scar tissue can also be decreased with injection of the chemotherapeutic drug 5-fluorouracil (5-FU). Intralesional injection of 5-FU improves the appearance of proliferative scars and decreases the chance of recurrence. 5-FU is most effective when used in combination with adjuvant therapy such as low-dose corticosteroids.[38]

- Hyperpigmentation may improve over time with sun avoidance. Topical hydroquinone gel may aid in preventing permanent scar discoloration.
- Dermabrasion, laser treatments, or chemical resurfacing may also be considered 6 weeks after the primary surgery when scars are persistently uneven.
- Ultimately scar excision and closure with multiple Z-plasties may be considered once healed in cases of forehead or cheek flaps.[24]

### Revision

- The ultimate option for the management of complications following nasal reconstruction is revision. Menick (2012) determines the type of revision indicated by considering: "1. The original goal of repair, 2. The defect site, size, and depth, 3. The availability and choice of donor materials, methods, and surgical stages, 4. Patient factors, and 5. Unforeseen problems."[6] Complex nasal reconstruction may require revision to re-establish nasal form and function, which can be defined as minor revision, major revision, or reoperation:[8]
  - Minor revision: Essential quality, outline, and contour restored with inadequate landmark definition.
  - Major revision: Failure of dimension, volume, contour, and symmetry or function.
  - Reoperation: Cover and lining grossly deficient. Normal must be returned to normal and the repair redone with a second regional flap."[8]

### Flap refinement

- Flap refinement is frequently indicated in nasal reconstruction, sculpting the subcutaneous tissue to enhance the ultimate esthetic outcome.
- Flap refinement may take place at the time of initial repair; however, there may be limits to the extent of thinning and debulking. Additional flap sculpting can be in stages, typically at 3-month intervals.
- Patient factors may influence the timing of flap refinement. For example, in smokers, the preference would be for delayed refinement.
- Pincushion deformities can be prevented with wide-undermining and managed with primary subcutaneous debulking/thinning of the flap or additional staged procedures.[24,37]

## SUMMARY

- Nasal reconstruction is a complex process that involves significant planning. Through anticipation of potential complications that may arise in the preoperative, intraoperative, or postoperative settings, surgeons may adjust practices and enhance outcomes.

- In the preoperative setting, thorough medical history taking, including patient comorbidities and medication and/or supplement use, is necessary to optimize outcomes. Notably, smoking cessation and improved glucose control are areas of preoperative optimization that have a significant impact on wound healing.
- Intraoperatively, emphasis on surgical technique principles, such as tension-free wound closure, hemostasis, and precise flap design, prevents complications.
- Through close perioperative wound care, adjunct therapies, and identification of need for revision, surgeons can prevent and manage complications effectively postoperatively.

## CLINICS CARE POINTS

- Prevention of complications in nasal reconstruction starts in the preoperative setting. Patient-specific factors can be optimized prior to intervention. Smoking cessation, tight blood glucose control in patients with diabetes, and holding anticoagulation medications/supplements are modifiable patient factors with significant impact on outcomes. Through close preoperative counseling and proactive management of modifiable risks, complications may be prevented.

- Intraoperatively, surgical technique combined with anticipation of flap-specific challenges allow for surgeons to avoid common complications. Maintenance of sterile surgical field and obeying key surgical tenants such as tension-free closure, hemostasis, and respect for nasal and facial subunits, aids in preventing complications.

- In the postoperative setting, close follow-up allows for early identification of complications. Effective management of complications is founded in vigilant wound care, adjunct therapies, and potential additional procedures. Patients should be appropriately counseled that nasal reconstruction is a complex process that frequently requires a staged plan of repair.

## DISCLOSURE

There are no commercial or financial conflicts of interest and any funding sources for all authors.

## REFERENCES

1. Borsuk DE, Papanastasiou C, Chollet A. Fine Details That Improve Nasal Reconstruction. Plast Reconstr Surg 2021;148:634e–44e.
2. Nesemeier R, Dunlap N, McClave SA, et al. Evidence-Based Support for Nutrition Therapy in Head and Neck Cancer. Curr Surg Rep 2017;5:18.
3. Grada A, Phillips TJ. Nutrition and cutaneous wound healing. Clin Dermatol 2022;40:103–13.
4. Owusu J, Nesbitt B, Boahene K. Management of Complicated Nasal Defects. Facial Plast Surg 2020;36:158–65.
5. Wu SS, Patel V, Oladeji T, et al. Development of a Risk Prediction Model for Complications Following Forehead Flaps for Nasal and Periorbital Reconstruction. J Craniofac Surg 2023;34:362–7.
6. Menick FJ. An approach to the late revision of a failed nasal reconstruction. Plast Reconstr Surg 2012;129:92e–103e.
7. Jewett BS. CHAPTER 26 - Complications of local flaps. In: Baker SR, editor. Local flaps in facial reconstruction. 2nd edition. Philadelphia, PA: Mosby; 2007. p. 691–722.
8. Menick FJ. Nasal reconstruction. Plast Reconstr Surg 2010;125:138e–50e.
9. Little SC, Hughley BB, Park SS. Complications with forehead flaps in nasal reconstruction. Laryngoscope 2009;119:1093–9.
10. Fulcher SM, Koman LA, Smith BP, et al. The effect of transdermal nicotine on digital perfusion in reformed habitual smokers. J Hand Surg Am 1998;23:792–9.
11. Nolan MB, Warner DO. Safety and Efficacy of Nicotine Replacement Therapy in the Perioperative Period: A Narrative Review. Mayo Clin Proc 2015; 90:1553–61.
12. Sorensen LT. Wound healing and infection in surgery: the pathophysiological impact of smoking, smoking cessation, and nicotine replacement therapy: a systematic review. Ann Surg 2012;255:1069–79.
13. Hatfield J, Saad S, Housewright C. Dietary supplements and bleeding. SAVE Proc 2022;35:802–7.
14. Wang CZ, Moss J, Yuan CS. Commonly Used Dietary Supplements on Coagulation Function during Surgery. Medicines (Basel) 2015;2:157–85.
15. Deirdre S, Leake SRB. CHAPTER 27 - Scar revision and local flap refinement. In: Baker SR, editor. Local flaps in facial reconstruction. 2nd edition. Mosby; 2007. p. 723–60.
16. Griffin GR, Chepeha DB, Moyer JS. Interpolated subcutaneous fat pedicle melolabial flap for large nasal lining defects. Laryngoscope 2013;123:356–9.
17. Kline RM. Aesthetic reconstruction of the nose following skin cancer. Clin Plast Surg 2004;31: 93–111.
18. Dronge AS, Perkal MF, Kancir S, et al. Long-term glycemic control and postoperative infectious

complications. Arch Surg 2006;141:375–80. discussion 380.

19. Kaplan AL, Cook JL. The incidences of chondritis and perichondritis associated with the surgical manipulation of auricular cartilage. Dermatol Surg 2004;30:58–62. discussion 62.

20. Weber SM, Baker SR. Management of cutaneous nasal defects. Facial Plast Surg Clin North Am 2009;17:395–417.

21. Bloom JD, Ransom ER, Miller CJ. Reconstruction of alar defects. Facial Plast Surg Clin North Am 2011; 19:63–83.

22. Menick FJ. Forehead flap: master techniques in otolaryngology-head and neck surgery. Facial Plast Surg 2014;30:131–44.

23. Correa BJ, Weathers WM, Wolfswinkel EM, et al. The forehead flap: the gold standard of nasal soft tissue reconstruction. Semin Plast Surg 2013;27:96–103.

24. Dibelius GS, Toriumi DM. Reconstruction of Cutaneous Nasal Defects. Facial Plast Surg Clin North Am 2017;25:409–26.

25. Stavrou D, Weissman O, Winkler E, et al. Silicone-based scar therapy: a review of the literature. Aesthetic Plast Surg 2010;34:646–51.

26. Yamasaki A, Dermody SM, Moyer JS. Reducing Risks of Graft Failure for Composite Skin-Cartilage Grafts. Facial Plast Surg Clin North Am 2023;31: 289–96.

27. Aden KK, Biel MA. The evaluation of pharmacologic agents on composite graft survival. Arch Otolaryngol Head Neck Surg 1992;118:175–8.

28. Kerolus JL, Nassif PS. Treatment Protocol for Compromised Nasal Skin. Facial Plast Surg Clin North Am 2019;27:505–11.

29. Wang W, Ong A, Vincent AG, et al. Flap Failure and Salvage in Head and Neck Reconstruction. Semin Plast Surg 2020;34:314–20.

30. Conforti ML, Connor NP, Heisey DM, et al. Evaluation of performance characteristics of the medicinal leech (Hirudo medicinalis) for the treatment of venous congestion. Plast Reconstr Surg 2002;109: 228–35.

31. Harun A, Kruer RM, Lee A, et al. Experience with pharmacologic leeching with bivalirudin for adjunct treatment of venous congestion of head and neck reconstructive flaps. Microsurgery 2018;38:643–50.

32. Li EN, Menon NG, Rodriguez ED, et al. The effect of hyperbaric oxygen therapy on composite graft survival. Ann Plast Surg 2004;53:141–5.

33. Sonker A, Dubey A, Bhatnagar A, et al. Platelet growth factors from allogeneic platelet-rich plasma for clinical improvement in split-thickness skin graft. Asian J Transfus Sci 2015;9:155–8.

34. Sommeling CE, Heyneman A, Hoeksema H, et al. The use of platelet-rich plasma in plastic surgery: a systematic review. J Plast Reconstr Aesthetic Surg 2013;66:301–11.

35. Frautschi RS, Hashem AM, Halasa B, et al. Current Evidence for Clinical Efficacy of Platelet Rich Plasma in Aesthetic Surgery: A Systematic Review. Aesthetic Surg J 2017;37:353–62.

36. San-Marina S, Sharma A, Voss SG, et al. Assessment of Scaffolding Properties for Chondrogenic Differentiation of Adipose-Derived Mesenchymal Stem Cells in Nasal Reconstruction. JAMA Facial Plast Surg 2017;19:108–14.

37. Sharma A, Janus JR, Hamilton GS. Regenerative medicine and nasal surgery. Mayo Clin Proc 2015; 90:148–58.

38. Shah VV, Aldahan AS, Mlacker S, et al. 5-Fluorouracil in the Treatment of Keloids and Hypertrophic Scars: A Comprehensive Review of the Literature. Dermatol Ther 2016;6:169–83.

# Management of Traumatic Nasal Avulsion Injuries

Scott Bevans, MD

## KEYWORDS

• Nasal avulsion • Nasal amputation • Replantation • Nasal reconstruction

## KEY POINTS

- Decontamination with dilute betadine and saline with preservation of vascular supply is paramount in partial avulsion injuries.
- For total avulsion injuries, tissue cooling with replantation within 12 hours provides optimal outcomes with single-stage surgery. While this can be technically demanding, even single artery anastomosis can result in near-full tissue survival.
- When staged reconstruction is anticipated, preserving cartilage and some tissue can be accomplished with tissue replacement, while preventing infection with appropriate antimicrobial coverage.

## INTRODUCTION

In any reconstructive surgery, the premise of "replace like with like" offers the best esthetic and functional outcome. This is particularly true of facial reconstructive surgery. The nose is a prominent portion of our midfacial identity. Recall that the loss of functional oral and nasal subunits has been considered the minimal indication for facial transplantation to offer patients a return to function within society.[1] In cases of traumatic nasal amputation injuries, replacing the avulsed nasal tissue has the potential to provide the best optimal functional and cosmetic consequences assuming vascular supply is adequate to sustain healing functions.

### Nature of Avulsive Nasal Injuries

Exact data on the frequency of avulsive midfacial soft tissue injuriesare complex to extract. A retrospective review of emergency room visits in 2011 found that 5 million visits were related to head and neck trauma, with over 40% of patients having an open wound.[2] The mechanism for these injuries may be blunt trauma, motor vehicle trauma, industrial machinery incidents, violence, or bite-related traumatic avulsions. While bite injuries are not the most common cause of soft tissue injury, most of the reported total nasal avulsion injuries from the last 20 years have been secondary to canine bites, particularly true in children.[3–5]

### History of Nasal Replantation

In the early 1970s multiple case reports were published about non-microvascular replantation of avulsed nasal soft tissues.[6] The traditional dogma was tissue must be replaced within 2 hours of avulsion or the prognosis for survival was "dismal."[7] Even under ideal circumstances, the best outcomes achieved typically still had partial soft tissue loss but with minimal contraction, creating a healthy wound bed that would accommodate skin grafting within a few weeks.[7]

In 1976, Norman James[8] published the first case of a successfully replanted avulsed lip and nasal injury using microvascular anastomosis.

Over the past 5 decades, advances in techniques, visualization, and applications of microsurgical techniques have led to the replantation of multiple facial subunit avulsion injuries.[9] The results in many of these patients would have required multiple staged surgical procedures to rebuild large cutaneous defects, often with complex composite defects in the lower one-third of the nose. Conversely, a single-stage replantation has the potential to restore the entire soft tissue envelope and cartilaginous structures. For surgeons who have performed replantation, the

Department of Otolaryngology, Tripler Army Medical Center, 1 Jarrett White Road, TAMC, HI 96818, USA
E-mail address: scott.e.bevans.mil@health.mil

Facial Plast Surg Clin N Am 32 (2024) 315–325
https://doi.org/10.1016/j.fsc.2024.01.007
1064-7406/24/Published by Elsevier Inc.

facialplastic.theclinics.com

restoration of viability to large composite tissue allografts seems nearly miraculous, and outcomes can be exceedingly favorable. Critics observe that microvascular replantation is time-sensitive, carries some technical complexity, and requires a longer immediate postoperative inpatient observation. However, given the excellent functional and cosmetic results achievable with replantation, proponents argue that particularly in larger, complex defects, an attempt should be made to replant, assuming capable surgical abilities and a feasible timeline.

## GENERAL APPROACH
### Trauma Patient Management

The approach to any trauma patient should be in accordance with advanced trauma life support protocols using primary and secondary surveys to identify and treat life-threatening injuries. In cases of nasal trauma, careful evaluation of surrounding structures including ocular, oral cavity, and adjacent nerve injuries is warranted. Limiting blood entering the nasal airway is necessary ideally without cauterizing wound edges. Identification of any other injuries that would preclude a multiple-hour surgical intervention is necessary if replantation is going to be considered, including attention to cervical spine clearance and screening for cranial injuries.

Blood loss can be significant in midface avulsion injuries, particularly when limiting hemostasis to facilitate replantation. Patients should be adequately resuscitated and typed and crossed for blood transfusions.

Importantly, facial skeleton injuries in the immediate area must be treated prior to replantation or tissue replacement to limit tension on the soft tissue repair, neurorrhaphy, and/or anastomosis. To facilitate identification and treatment planning, physicians should have a low threshold to obtain a fine-cut maxillofacial computed tomography scan.

### Decontamination and Wound Bed Preparation

For decontaminating wounds in awake patients, consider regional blocks (infraorbital nerve, infratrochlear nerve, external nasal nerve) to avoid injection of hemostatic agents directly into the wound edge.

The military's recently updated Joint Trauma System Clinical Practice Guideline for the treatment of traumatic soft tissue wounds recommends low-pressure irrigation of 1 to 3 L for small wounds, with increasing volumes for larger wounds. Pressurized irrigation systems did not reduce the risk of infection, and some studies raised concerns about seeding bacterial contaminants deeper in the wound or along fascial planes.[10] While large open wounds may not benefit from wound cleansers over normal saline alone, studies of smaller or closed wounds show a decreased infection rate when using a mild cleanser (1%–10% iodine). Therefore, most investigators recommend at least cleansing avulsed tissue (particularly with exposed cartilage) using 10% povidone-iodine and saline.[11]

Wound bed debridement should be performed with warm saline after decontamination. Gentle tissue handling with detailed attention to vascular sources is recommended as vasodilation that occurs with warm irrigation may facilitate identifying spasmed vessels that may be preserved (in partial avulsions) used for anastomosis (in total avulsion injuries).

### Antimicrobial Prophylaxis

As with all soft tissue injuries, appropriate tetanus prophylaxis should be employed. With bite wounds, indications for rabies prophylaxis should be considered. Tailored antimicrobial therapy is likely warranted based on the mechanism of injury. For canine bite wounds, the most common and virulent cause of infection in the first 24 hours is *Pasteurella multocida*, which can cause a significant inflammatory response, rapidly progressive infection, and necrosis.[3] The second most common organism is *Capnocytophaga canimorsus*.[12] Delayed infections are more commonly secondary to *Staphylococcus* and *Streptococcus*. Fortunately, prophylaxis with amoxicillin with clavulanic acid, or tetracycline or doxycycline with metronidazole in penicillin-allergic patients generally covers all these pathogens appropriately.[3] Human bite wounds tend to transmit even more bacterial load to the victim; however, bacteriology in human bite wounds is largely *Streptococcus*, *Staphylococcus*, and *Eikenella corrodens*.[12] Although *Staphylococcus aureus* is the most common identified etiology for nasal cartilage infection, in cartilage-exposed avulsion injuries, consideration may be given to coverage for *Pseudomonas aeruginosa* infections.[13–15]

## PARTIAL NASAL AVULSION INJURIES
### Preserving Partially Avulsed Tissue

In the initial evaluation, preservation of any soft tissue connection is advised. **Fig. 1**A demonstrates a subtotal avulsion injury in a pediatric patient from a dog bite. As is often the case in subtotal avulsion injuries, only a single arterial inflow remains (left angular artery in the case demonstrated). Despite this relatively limited arterial inflow, the majority of the tissue was preserved secondary to the

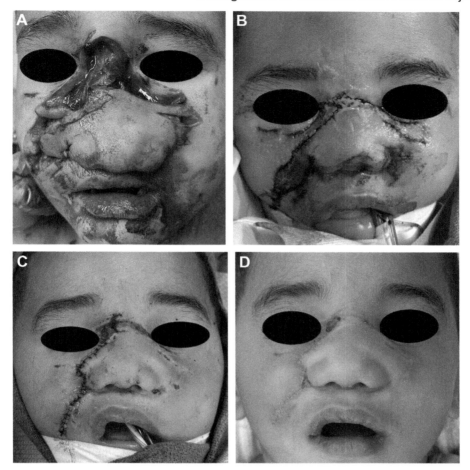

**Fig. 1.** A pediatric patient with incomplete nasal avulsion injury from a dog bite injury. (*A*) The remaining vascular pedicle is on the patient's left side. Arterial supply to the right aspect of the wound was entirely disrupted. The patient was placed on weight-based aspirin, with abrasion and heparin-soaked gauze treatment to the right nasofacial aspect of the replaced graft. (*B*) Despite the small amount of remaining vascular inflow, most of the tissue survived. (*C*) At 1 week and with resection of the devitalized tissue on the right aspect of the wound. (*D*) One week after revision, an excellent functional and esthetic result was achieved. (*Courtesy of* Dr Patrick O'Donnell, MD.)

generous vascular collateralization in the nose. As in other case reports of large nasal avulsions with only a single intact arterial inflow, excellent healing potential is possible. (**Fig. 1**D).

Evaluation may be most effective under general anesthesia and infiltration of local anesthetic using only regional blocks (without epinephrine) which may additionally promote sympathetic block and potential vasodilation.[16] During this phase, care should be taken not to traumatize or compress the remaining pedicle of tissue. Running sutures may.

As with other microvascular techniques, perfusion assessment can be performed with a 25-gauge or 27-gauge needle stick and/or capillary refill. The use of intravenous (IV) indocyanine green provides additional visualization of angiosomes. Only conservative resection of potentially viable tissue should be considered.

### Wound Closure

Shearing forces on the replanted segment during healing will disrupt the angiogenesis process. Many of these injuries are prone to contamination and buried sutures may increase the risk of infection. Running sutures may restrict blood flow at the wound edge. Thus, interrupted monofilament sutures (avoiding the anastomosis) are the preferred method for closure.

### Postoperative Care

Surgeons will still likely need to consider therapies to avoid venous congestion, including 2 leeches every 6 hours for 48 hours, needle sticks every 4 hours for venous drainage, or heparin gauze scrubs.[16–18] (See the following "*Addressing Venous Congestion*" sectionfor additional details.) The tissue should be kept moist and clean. Under the best circumstances, some amount of soft tissue loss should be anticipated, and revision surgery should be anticipated in the first 2 weeks after injury (**Fig. 1**B and C). In cases of more significant progressive soft tissue loss, hyperbaric oxygen (HBO) may be considered (See the following "Hyperbaric Oxygen Therapy" section).

## COMPLETE NASAL AVULSION INJURIES
### How to Preserve Completely Avulsed Tissue

Ideal tissue handling lowers the metabolic demand while preventing cold burns from direct contact with ice. Expert consensus recommends storage as close as possible to 4°C by wrapping avulsed tissue in dry gauze, placing it in a leak-proof plastic bag and placing it on ice.[19]

### Treatment Options

Four broad options exist for the treatment of full avulsion injuries: (1) microvascular replantation, (2) tissue replacement without revascularization, (3) immediate regional reconstruction, or (4) wound stabilization for delayed reconstruction.

In patients with concomitant facial skeleton trauma, appropriate reduction and fixation should generally be performed before attempts at tissue replacement or revascularization to avoid tension on the wound edges and/or vascular pedicle. In cases of incomplete avulsion injuries, excellent outcomes can be achieved by preserving even single sources of arterial supply due to the generous collateralization of the midface vasculature. Advocates for replantation in full avulsion injuries argue that the benefits of replantation from a functional and esthetic standpoint are so advantageous (particularly in complex injuries) given the capabilities for the microvascular repair and lack of significant comorbidities precluding an operative intervention, that an attempt at replantation should be made.

### Microvascular replantation
While technical complexity can be high, there have been many successful reports of replantation in various facial subunits, including nasal tissue, ear, lip, cheek, and scalp.

Small anastomoses (in many cases requiring "super-microsurgery"), relatively low-flow states, direct and indirect vessel injury, and overall coagulopathies all predispose to thrombosis. With the elevated risk of thrombosis, systemic and local anticoagulation techniques are employed. Because it is more commonly performed in extremities, many of the dosing regimens and techniques for facial subunit replantation techniques are borrowed from extremity replantation protocols.

Many outcomes of replantation show excellent cosmetic results, with fewer than 30% requiring additional surgeries.[9] Interestingly, sensory outcomes in many patients were excellent, with a full return of sensory function.[20]

As this is an uncommonly performed procedure for even experienced microvascular surgeons, on-line and telephone replantation guidelines are available through the Buncke Microvascular Clinic, with an on-call attending physician for emergency consultation (Contact information available at: https://thebunckeclinic.org/replantation). Other online resources can be found through Web sites (free with registration) such as https://www.microsurgeon.org/replantation.

**Timeline for replantation** When appropriately cooled, case reports have demonstrated successful replantation of auricular avulsion injuries as late as 33 hours after injury when tissue is preserved in this fashion.[21] In nasal injuries specifically, the maximum reported cold ischemia time reported with a successful outcome is 13 hours.[22]

The duration of operative intervention ranges from 1.5 to 10 hours depending on additional injuries, with most reporting 7+ hours for surgery.[17,23] Therefore, any patient presenting with a properly preserved avulsed tissue segment within 12 to 18 hours of injury may potentially be a viable candidate for replantation.

**Contraindications for replantation** When tissue is severely crushed or has multiple lacerations that disrupt blood flow in the avulsed segment, revascularization is less likely to be successful. Tissue with prolonged ischemia times or inappropriate preservation is more likely to be thrombogenic and less likely to reperfuse well. However, until an attempt at reperfusion is made, the capacity for vascular flow may not be known.

Patients with religious exceptions to blood transfusion may not be candidates.

Patients with comorbidities or injuries that would preclude a (potentially) prolonged general anesthetic and/or anticoagulation are poor candidates for attempted replantation.

**Technical aspects**
*Identifying vessels in the avulsed tissue* Identifying vessels in the avulsed tissue is possible with loupe magnification, but it is easiest under the microscope. This can be accomplished while the patient is still being anesthetized. When identified, gentle cannulation and irrigation with heparinized saline can help dilate the vessels. Microvascular Acland clamps can then be used as markers.

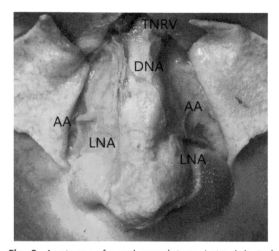

**Fig. 2.** Anatomy of nasal vasculature. Latex-injected cadaveric dissection demonstrating the location and relative diameter of the angular artery (AA), lateral nasal artery (LNA), and dorsal nasal artery (DNA). Note the variation in course but consistent depth (just superficial to the perichondrium/periosteum). Also, note the confluence of the smaller dorsal nasal veins in the transverse and characteristically larger vein, referred to as the "transverse nasal root vein" (TNRV) that continues superiorly through the glabella. (*Reprinted from* Sykes, J. M., & Bray, H. N. (2022). Understanding the Vascular Anatomy of the Face: Introducing the X-Y-Z-Concept. *Facial Plast Surg Clin North Am*, 30(2), 233-237.)

Avulsed vessels (particularly veins) often have intimal injuries or tears which may require resection beyond the zone of trauma.

**Finding donor vessels** The perinasal arteries measure between 0.5 and 1.5 mm.[24] Angular, dorsal nasal, lateral nasal, supratrochlear, and superior labial arteries have all been used for arterial anastomosis.[9,25] The location of the angular artery is consistent, while that of the dorsal nasal artery and lateral nasal artery may be variable in course but consistent in depth (**Fig. 2**).[26] Anterior ethmoid arteries (on the internal side of the nasal bones and cartilage) have also been used.[27] For larger arterial access, the proximal portion of the angular artery or the facial artery must be utilized. Reaching larger caliber vessels such as the facial artery and facial vein will undoubtedly require interposition grafts in isolated nasal avulsion injuries.

Venous anastomosis has been more frequently reported in the angular and infratrochlear vessels (near the nasolabial fold or glabella, respectively).[9] On cadaveric venograms, there is often a confluence of the angular veins in the infratrochlear vein which travels transverse and then superiorly to join the supratrochlear system (see **Fig. 2**).

**Stabilization of avulsed tissue** Accurate orientation of the avulsed tissue may be helpful before attempting anastomosis. One or 2 cardinal sutures on a single edge of the tissue can still allow reflection of the tissue for access to vasculature. In full-thickness avulsion injuries, surgeons may consider repairing the internal lining to anchor the graft. While precise reapproximation of the wound edges must follow microvascular anastomosis, insetting the avulsed tissue before anastomosis will confirm if interposition grafts will be necessary. Once re-anastomosis is performed, the tissue can become engorged and edematous, making stabilization of the anastomosis difficult with larger segments.

**Using interposition grafts** For either or both arterial and venous anastomosis, interposition grafts are frequently required to reach beyond the zone of injury (**Fig. 3**). Donor sites have been described from the superficial temporal veins and superficial arm or foot veins.[25,28-30]

Standard microsurgical techniques can be used if the diameter of the vessels allows. Particularly, in the case of interposition grafts, addressing diameter mismatch may be required. Several well-described techniques exist to taper vessel diameter by excising a corner of the larger diameter vessel and oversewing it.[31]

**Tips for performing anastomosis** Super-microsurgery is defined as surgical anastomosis of vessels smaller than 1 mm. Multiple investigators have described anastomosing sub-millimeter vessels in pediatric and/or small tissue defects. Investigators with experience in these techniques advocate for 10-0 or 11-0 nylon sutures in cardinal positions (4 in total).[32] Additional puncture sites in small vessel walls may increase the potential for thrombosis and/or back-walling the vessel.

The venous outflow from the avulsed segment may not be as visible until the arterial flow is established. When possible, vein to vein anastomosis should be performed. If suitable donor veins cannot be identified to complete the anastomosis, case reports have shown that sewing an artery to a vein (creating a fistula) has been effective.[9]

There are several case reports describing nasal avulsion injuries that have been treated with arterial-only anastomosis.[9,33] However, the larger the avulsed segment, the more important the venous anastomosis. Venous thrombosis has been reported and corrected with exploration.[9,25]

**Addressing venous congestion** Even without thrombosis of the anastomosis, venous congestion is common.[9] Neovascularization can begin rapidly (some authors estimate angiogenesis

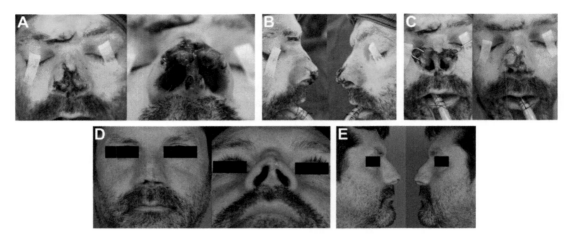

**Fig. 3.** A middle-aged male with a partial nasal tip avulsion injury from scraping the asphalt during a motorcycle accident. (*A*) Initial injury frontal and base views. (*B*) Lateral views demonstrate the soft tissue loss in the tip and infratip. (*C*) Cartilage and intranasal injury with final closure of lacerations. The resulting defect was covered with acellular dermal replacement. (*D*) One year after repair without additional revision patient declined further treatment for nasal tip deformity. (*E*). Lateral views, 1 year after injury. (Photos courtesy of Sam Oyer, MD.)

within 48 hours). However, until this occurs, the mechanisms for treating venous congestion are largely mechanical drainage of excess blood from the tissue through tissue disruption and prevention of clot formation.

One of the oldest techniques to treat venous congestion is the use of medicinal leeches (hirudotherapy or therapy using *Hirudo medicinalis*). Leeches may need to be initiated in the operating room and may be required for a few or several days (one case report of a large lip and nasal avulsion injury describes using 358 leeches in the 14 days following surgery).[33] Common utilization is 2 leeches every 6 to 8 hours for 48 hours.[9,17] In pediatric patients, need for leech therapy may require general anesthesia. Coverage for *Aeromonas hydrophilia* with ciprofloxacin is necessary when using leech therapy. Scarring from leech therapy is rare but has been reported after healing.[9]

Several alternatives to hirudotherapy can also be employed.

- Heparin-soaked gauze with needle sticks performed every 4 hours.[9]
- Heparin gauze scrubs every 3 to 6 hours.[17]
- Direct injection of low-molecular-weight heparin (LMWH) into the graft with sponge abrasion.[34]
- Continuous heparinized irrigation through a drain tube for 1 week (concentration of 12,500 units of heparin in 250 mL of normal saline).[35]

Most investigators report venous congestion begins to improve by postoperative days 3 to 6 but can last significantly longer depending on the size of the replanted tissue and the number of venous anastomoses.[17,25,33,34]

***Use of systemic anticoagulation*** Secondary to the high thrombogenic potential and small vasculature, most advocate for a loading dose of anticoagulation as well as layered postoperative therapy.

*Heparin/low-molecular-weight heparin* Intraoperative loading dose protocols for factor Xa inhibitors during replantation range from a simple 5000 unit bolus[25] to 50 units/kg.[36,37] IV heparin is often continued for at least 36 hours, with a goal of 1.5 times normal partial thromboplastin time.[25] Acute coronary syndrome dosing is generally unnecessary, although titration to the endpoint of perfusion is advised.[38]

LMWH can be alternatively used at a dose of 5000 units twice a day.[33] A Cochrane review comparing unfractionated heparin with LMWH found no difference in vessel thrombosis rates in digit replants but fewer complications with LMWH.[37]

***Dextran*** Some protocols advocate for the addition of dextran to protect vessel patency (coating the endothelium, binding platelets, and red blood cells). Dextran 40 is commonly used at 25 mL per hour (8 mL/kg/24 hours in children). Although rare, pulmonary edema may result.[39]

***Aspirin*** Aspirin (325 mg) is commonly used and effective in preventing thrombosis in microvascular surgery.[33] In children, dosing is less (80 mg) and care should be taken to avoid Reye syndrome.[38]

**Topical agents** Other adjuncts are topical lidocaine, papaverine (both smooth muscle relaxants), and nitroglycerin paste (vasodilator).[9]

**Blood transfusions** Likely secondary to these measures to prevent thrombosis, persistent bleeding resulting in the need for transfusion is common. Williams and colleagues[9] reported that among case reports of facial subunit replantation following dog bite injuries, more than 80% required transfusions. While these injuries included several larger areas of tissue loss, care teams should be prepared for the potential of prolonged blood loss.

**Wound closure** Similar to partial nasal avulsion injuries, closure adequate to prevent shearing forces on the replanted segment will prevent disrupting angiogenesis. Minimal buried sutures should be employed, and interrupted monofilament sutures (avoiding the anastomosis) are preferred over running sutures.

**Postoperative care** As with all free tissue transfer, regular assessment of the arterial and venous flow should be performed according to preferred protocols. The tissue should be kept moist and clean. Under the ideal reperfusion results, approximately 30% of patients will still develop partial (often superficial) tissue loss requiring debridement or minor scar revision.[9] When considering the approach for addressing scar contracture, time since replantation, location of the pedicle, and approach must be considered, as even a traditionally well-tolerated open rhinoplasty approach may be contraindicated based on the location of anastomosis.[40]

### Tissue replacement without microvascular anastomosis

Even when microvascular replantation is not feasible in fully avulsed tissue, some benefits may exist from the replacement of tissue. Particularly for small-volume full tissue avulsions (less than 1.5 cm$^2$), relatively rapid angiogenesis may allow for the preservation of at least internal lining and cartilaginous structures.[20]

**Re-suturing completely avulsed tissue** Before the development of microvascular replantation techniques, avulsed tissue was commonly sewn directly back into the wound. Retrospective reviews have demonstrated that the volume and composition of tissue, as well as pre-morbid factors related to the potential for revascularization, are predictive of the ability for tissue survival. Specifically, a tissue area less than 1.5 cm$^2$, when placed into a healthy vascular bed has a reasonable chance of at least partial survival.[6,20] This

technique is, in essence, using the avulsed tissue as a composite graft. Similar tenants of wound decontamination and tissue preservation (eg, cooling to lower metabolic demand) are still apropos. Here again, the graft should be inset with interrupted monofilament sutures (running sutures may constrict blood flow to the edge, and buried sutures may predispose to infection).

Despite the complete lack of arterial flow, some surgeons still attempt leech therapy to introduce oxygenation, particularly in cases of suspected early angiogenesis. Appropriate antibiotic therapy is warranted.

**Hyperbaric oxygen** In case reports using daily HBO for 7 to 12 days after non-vascularized replantation, none resulted a 100% survival; however, partial salvage was common, and the volume of tissue was possibly improved.[41,42]

**Postoperative care** The tissue should be kept moist and clean. The use of liberal topical antimicrobial ointment is common unless contraindicated by HBO or therapies targeting the prevention of venous congestion previously discussed (ie, leeches, heparin-soaked gauze scrubs, and so forth). Patients should be counseled to expect partial or superficial tissue loss requiring future debridement, scar revision, or adjacent tissue transfer. Weekly assessments of the tissue are likely warranted to recognize early infection and begin developing a shared surgical plan with patients for future interventions (**Fig. 4**).

### Immediate regional reconstruction

Traditional dogma in trauma injuries is to allow for wound declaration and stabilization before performing locoregional reconstruction. This paradigm was developed because of the tissue damage that accompanies significant blunt force or ballistic trauma.[11] However, often in nasal avulsion injuries specifically, the zone of injury to surrounding soft tissue may be relatively small. Recent advocates for immediate locoregional reconstruction (which is commonly a paramedian forehead flap) indicate that increased blood flow may decrease the degree of post-traumatic tissue loss.[43–45] While this remains an option, many surgeons delay regional reconstruction techniques for at least 1 to 4 weeks following the trauma.

### Wound stabilization for delayed reconstruction

When no tissue is available (or feasible) to replace, most surgeons will attempt to cover bone or cartilage with soft tissue (for example, closing the mucosa to the skin to prevent chronic exposure). When impractical, several acellular dermal replacement products are available as

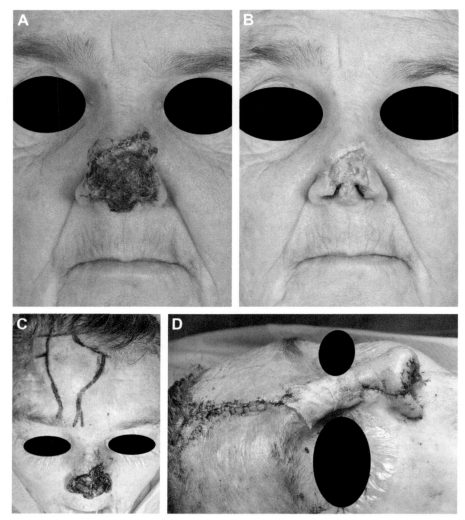

**Fig. 4.** A 60-year-old female with composite nasal tip avulsion injury. The tissue was re-sutured without microvascular replantation. (*A*) 1 week after injury. (*B*) Note partial survival of the internal lining and minimal cartilage at the time of delayed reconstruction 1 month after injury. (*C*) Pre-expanded paramedian forehead flap (PMFF) following cartilage reconstruction of the lower nasal third. (*D*) Following PMFF inset.

semipermeable wound dressings which can help preserve exposed cartilage and facilitate granulation tissue and re-epithelialization. **Fig. 3** demonstrates a nasal tip loss treated with primary closure of the nasal mucosa and remaining cartilage with an acellular dermal matrix allowing impressive healing potential before further surgery. When necessary, silicone tubing can be placed in the nasal apertures following avulsion injuries to prevent stenosis, maintain the nasal airway, and promote granulation bed formation for future mucosal/skin reconstruction.[46,47]

### Nonsurgical therapies: nasal prosthesis

In patients with total or sub-total nasal avulsion injuries that are not candidates for either

replantation or delayed surgical reconstruction, a skilled anaplastologist may be an invaluable resource. Nasal prosthetics can be challenging to manufacture, adhere, and color-match; however, for some patients, this may represent the lowest risk option for normal appearance. Details of nasal prostheses are discussed in the subsequent article of this publication.

### SUMMARY

In the "replace like with like" paradigm of facial reconstruction, there is no more exact replacement for nasal defect than the avulsed segment of tissue. If any remaining blood supply exists to the avulsed segment, replacement after fixation of skeletal injuries should be attempted. As replantation protocols become more common, early, appropriate tissue cooling is now more frequent, which can significantly improve the duration and therefore the opportunity for microvascular replantation. Although the vasculature seems dauntingly small, there are few better surgeons than those familiar both with the intricacies of facial vasculature anatomy and well-versed in microvascular techniques to successfully perform a replantation. Despite several practical hurdles, given the excellent esthetic and functional results, in healthy patients (and particularly children) with significant nasal avulsion injuries, an attempt at replantation should be entertained. Venous congestion in both partial and full avulsion injuries is common and multiple techniques can be employed to address this. When replacement of avulsed tissue is impossible, wound bed decontamination and remaining tissue preservation using biologic dressing options can be quite beneficial for definitive reconstruction or simply psychological preparation for future staged reconstruction.

## CLINICS CARE POINTS

- Nasal wound healing outcomes can be excellent by decontaminating and replacing large segment partial avulsion injuries that retain some vascular supply.

- Wound decontamination and atraumatic preparation are performed with low pressure, high-volume saline irrigation, and betadine.

- For complete amputation injuries to the nose, the best single-stage outcomes are achieved through microvascular tissue replantation, justifying an attempt at revascularization assuming access to surgeons with microvascular experience and/or availability.

- Completely avulsed tissue is ideally preserved at 4°C, which can be accomplished by wrapping it in gauze and placing it in a sealed plastic bag placed on ice.

- When ideally preserved, successful replantation can be performed several hours after injury.

- Single-artery anastomosis is usually adequate for tissue perfusion, although larger segments benefit significantly from venous anastomosis as well.

- Technical guides and 24-hour attending consultations are available through the Buncke microvascular clinic resources (https://thebunckeclinic.org/replantation).

- Venous congestion in both partial and full avulsion injuries is common and can be treated with several anticoagulation protocols (including IV heparin, subcutaneous LMWH, and antiplatelet agents) and/or leech therapy.

- In complete avulsion injuries, tissue replacement without an attempt at revascularization may have some benefit; however, except in small-volume tissue replacement, this technique will likely still require delayed reconstruction.

- HBOmay help increase the volume of tissue survival in non–re-vascularized tissue replantation.

## ACKNOWLEDGMENTS

The author wishes to thank: Dr Patrick McDonnell and Dr Samuel Oyer for providing photographs (with patient consent), as well as Dr Jonathan Sykes for the use of his excellent anatomic demonstration of nasal vasculature.

## DISCLOSURE

LTC S. Bevans is a member of the US Military. Reference herein to any specific commercial products, process, or service by trade name, trademark, manufacturer, or otherwise, does not necessarily constitute or imply its endorsement, recommendation, or favoring by the US Government. The views expressed here are those of the authors and do not reflect the official policy or position of the Department of the Army, Navy, Department of Defense, or the US Government. Financial Disclosures: None.

## REFERENCES

1. Alam DS, Chi JJ. Facial transplantation for massive traumatic injuries. Otolaryngol Clin North Am 2013; 46(5):883–901.
2. Sethi RK, Kozin ED, Fagenholz PJ, et al. Epidemiological survey of head and neck injuries and trauma in the United States. Otolaryngol Head Neck Surg 2014;151(5):776–84.
3. Morgan M, Palmer J. Dog bites. BMJ 2007; 334(7590):413–7.
4. Nathan JM, Ettinger KS. Management of Nasal Trauma. Oral Maxillofac Surg Clin North Am 2021; 33(3):329–41.
5. Mendoza JM, Chi JJ. Reconstruction of animal bite injuries to the head and neck. Curr Opin Otolaryngol Head Neck Surg 2019;27(5):407–12.

6. Grabb WC, Dingman RO. The fate of amputated tissues of the head and neck following replacement. Plast Reconstr Surg 1972;49(1):28–32.

7. Cort DF. Nasal tip replantation. case report. Plast Reconstr Surg 1973;52(2):194–6.

8. James NJ. Survival of large replanted segment of upper lip and nose. case report. Plast Reconstr Surg 1976;58(5):623–5.

9. Williams AJ, Powers JM, Rhodes JL, et al. Microvascular replantation following facial dog bites in children: systematic review and management algorithm. Ann Plast Surg 2018;81(1):106–12.

10. War wounds: debridement and irrigation (CPG ID: 31), Joint Trauma System Clinical Practice Guideline (JTS CPG). U.S. Defense Center of Excellence for Trauma; 2021.

11. Clark NW, Barrett DM, Kahmke RR, et al. Soft tissue trauma: critical recognition and timing of intervention in emergency presentations. Otolaryngol Clin North Am 2023;56(6):1003–12.

12. Rothe K, Tsokos M, Handrick W. Animal and human bite wounds. Dtsch Arztebl Int 2015;112(25): 433–42. quiz 443.

13. Zeng Q, Hu YG, Tang YX, et al. Complications and treatments of pseudomonas aeruginosa infection after rhinoplasty with implants: a clinical study. J Craniofac Surg 2023;34(2):e104–8.

14. Alshaikh N, Lo S. Nasal septal abscess in children: from diagnosis to management and prevention. Int J Pediatr Otorhinolaryngol 2011;75(6):737–44.

15. Close DM, Guinness MD. Abscess of the nasal septum after trauma. Med J Aust 1985;142(8): 472–4.

16. Pereira O, Bins-Ely J, Lobo GS, et al. Successful replantation of an almost-amputated nose. Plast Reconstr Surg 2010;125(6):249e–51e.

17. Kayikcioglu A, Karamursel S, Kecik A. Replantation of nearly total nose amputation without venous anastomosis. Plast Reconstr Surg 2001;108(3): 702–4.

18. Mortenson BW, Dawson KH, Murakami C. Medicinal leeches used to salvage a traumatic nasal flap. Br J Oral Maxillofac Surg 1998;36(6):462–4.

19. Lavasani L, Leventhal D, Constantinides M, et al. Management of acute soft tissue injury to the auricle. Facial Plast Surg 2010;26(6):445–50.

20. Marsden NJ, Kyle A, Jessop ZM, et al. Long-term outcomes of microsurgical nasal replantation: review of the literature and illustrated 10-year follow-up of a pediatric case with full sensory recovery. Front Surg 2015;2:6.

21. Shelley OP, Villafane O, Watson SB. Successful partial ear replantation after prolonged ischaemia time. Br J Plast Surg 2000;53(1):76–7.

22. Gilleard O, Smeets L, Seth R, et al. Successful delayed nose replantation following a dogbite: arterial and venous microanastomosis using interpositional vein grafts. J Plast Reconstr Aesthetic Surg 2014; 67(7):992–4.

23. Hussain G, Thomson S, Zielinski V. Nasal amputation due to human bite: microsurgical replantation. Aust N Z J Surg 1997;67(6):382–4.

24. Alfertshofer MG, Frank K, Moellhoff N, et al. Ultrasound anatomy of the dorsal nasal artery as it relates to liquid rhinoplasty procedures. Facial Plast Surg Clin North Am 2022;30(2):135–41.

25. Elzinga K, Medina A, Guilfoyle R. Total nose and upper lip replantation: a case report and literature review. Plast Reconstr Surg Glob Open 2018;6(10):e1839.

26. Sykes JM, Bray HN. Understanding the vascular anatomy of the face: introducing the X-Y-Z-concept. Facial Plast Surg Clin North Am 2022; 30(2):233–7.

27. Okumus A, Vasfi Kuvat S, Kabakas F. Successful replantation of an amputated nose after occupational injury. J Craniofac Surg 2010;21(1):289–90.

28. Hsieh YH, Medland J, Lin F, et al. Diversity of the free helical rim flap: a case series tailoring the microsurgical technique to esthetically optimize full-thickness nasal defect reconstructions. J Plast Reconstr Aesthetic Surg 2023;84:341–9.

29. Akyurek M, Perry D. Microsurgical replantation of completely avulsed nasal segment. J Craniofac Surg 2019;30(1):208–10.

30. Akyurek M, Safak T, Kecik A. Microsurgical revascularization of almost totally amputated alar wing of the nose. Ann Plast Surg 2004;53(2):181–4.

31. Zhang Y, Wang T, Liu Y, et al. Three end-to-end techniques for microvascular anastomosis of vessels with different size discrepancy. Ann Plast Surg 2020;85(2):141–5.

32. Tee R, Woodfield M. Supermicrosurgical replantation of a small amputated nasal tissue in a child. Clin Case Rep 2017;5(12):1961–5.

33. Larsson J, Klasson S, Arnljots B. Successful nose replantation using leeches for venous draining. Facial Plast Surg 2016;32(4):469–70.

34. Hammond DC, Bouwense CL, Hankins WT, et al. Microsurgical replantation of the amputated nose. Plast Reconstr Surg 2000;105(6):2133–6. quiz 2137; discussion 2138.

35. Yao JM, Yan S, Xu JH, et al. Replantation of amputated nose by microvascular anastomosis. Plast Reconstr Surg 1998;102(1):171–3.

36. Chen YC, Chan FC, Hsu CC, et al. Fingertip replantation without venous anastomosis. Ann Plast Surg 2013;70(3):284–8.

37. Chen YC, Chi CC, Chan FC, et al. Low molecular weight heparin for prevention of microvascular occlusion in digital replantation. Cochrane Database Syst Rev 2013;7:CD009894.

38. Buntic RF, Brooks D. Standardized protocol for artery-only fingertip replantation. J Hand Surg Am 2010;35(9):1491–6.

39. Buntic RF, Brooks D, Buncke HJ, et al. Dextran-related complications in head and neck microsurgery: do the benefits outweigh the risks? Plast Reconstr Surg 2004;114(4):1008. ; author reply 1008-1009.

40. Cooney DS, Fletcher DR, Bonawitz SC. Successful replantation of an amputated midfacial segment: technical details and lessons learned. Ann Plast Surg 2013;70(6):663–5.

41. Cantarella G, Mazzola RF, Pagani D. The fate of an amputated nose after replantation. Am J Otolaryngol 2005;26(5):344–7.

42. Pou JD, Graham HD. Pediatric nasal tip amputation successfully treated with nonmicrovascular replantation and hyperbaric oxygen therapy. Ochsner J 2017;17(2):204–7.

43. Ahmadi Moghadam M, Ahmadi Moghadam S. Use of forehead flap for nasal tip reconstruction after traumatic nasal amputation. World J Plast Surg 2017;6(3):361–4.

44. Shipkov H, Traikova N, Stefanova P, et al. The forehead flap for immediate reconstruction of the nose after bite injuries: indications, advantages, and disadvantages. Ann Plast Surg 2014;73(3):358.

45. Ramachandra T, Ries WR. Management of nasal and perinasal soft tissue injuries. Facial Plast Surg 2015;31(3):194–200.

46. Welch JA, Swaim SF. Nasal and facial reconstruction in a dog following severe trauma. J Am Anim Hosp Assoc 2003;39(4):407–15.

47. Kalmar CL, Nguyen PD, Taylor JA. Subtotal nasal reconstruction after traumatic avulsion. Plast Reconstr Surg Glob Open 2020;8(11):e3239.

# Prosthetic Nasal Reconstruction

Michelle K. Ruse, DDS, MDS[a], Michaela Calhoun, MS, CCA[b], Betsy K. Davis, DMD, MS[a],*

## KEYWORDS

- Nasal prosthesis • Facial prosthesis • Maxillofacial prosthodontics • Maxillofacial rehabilitation
- Nasal defect • Nasal reconstruction • Rhinectomy

## KEY POINTS

- Nasal defects can result from surgical tumor removal, trauma, or congenital conditions.
- A nasal prosthesis can be used alone or in conjunction with surgical reconstruction and can serve as an interim or definitive treatment. Nasal prostheses function by restoring form to the external nose, protecting exposed mucosa and sensitive tissue, supporting eyeglasses, and normalizing breathing and speech patterns. They improve patient esthetics, psychosocial well-being, and quality of life. Nasal prostheses require multidisciplinary care.
- Successful surgical reconstruction is dependent on patient factors like smoking and systemic health, along with the experience and skill of the surgeon. If surgical reconstruction is unlikely to provide a good esthetic and functional outcome, a prosthesis is recommended.
- Intentional surgical techniques and proper preparation of the defect can greatly influence the success of the nasal prosthetic rehabilitation. This may include removal of healthy hard and soft tissues. Collaboration between surgeons, maxillofacial prosthodontists and anaplastologists is the key.
- Creating realistic expectations with thorough patient education is critical for successful nasal prosthetic treatment.

## INTRODUCTION

The nose is a prominent central landmark on the face. Individuals seeking prosthetic nasal reconstruction may be missing nasal anatomy due to a traumatic injury, congenital malformation, or complications from an infection, but the most common cause of rhinectomy is tumor resection.[1,2] Head and neck cancer is the 7th most common cancer worldwide, with the majority of cases being squamous cell carcinomas. Head and neck cancer claims approximately 325,000 lives annually; the incidence is expected to increase.[3] Those who live with the aftermath of head and neck cancer can be left with extremely disfiguring defects that affect quality of life and the ability to work and socialize with friends and family. These devastating facial defects can also impede speech, mastication, and oral function.[1,2]

Nasal anatomy is a complex and delicate arrangement of layers of skin, cartilage, bone and mucosa.[4,5] Nasal defects can involve both intraoral and extraoral tissue, and the success of a total nasal surgical reconstruction is dependent upon the anatomic deficits, the health of the patient, and the skill of the surgeon. Surgical reconstruction is extremely complex with regard to anatomy, esthetics, and functional breathing,[4,6] and is not always the best option for restoring optimum esthetics and patient function.[1]

Nasal prostheses can restore esthetics and reproduce normal contours of the external nose, which functions in many ways for patients.[1,2,7] A nasal prosthesis protects exposed mucosa and

[a] HCA Healthcare and Sarah Cannon Cancer Institute, 9228 Medical Plaza Drive, Charleston, SC 29406, USA;
[b] Medical Art Resources, Inc and Prosthetics at Graphica Medica, 1880 Livingston Avenue, West Saint Paul, MN 55118, USA
* Corresponding author. 9228 Medical Plaza Drive, Charleston, SC 29406.
*E-mail address:* davisdkb@icloud.com

Facial Plast Surg Clin N Am 32 (2024) 327–337
https://doi.org/10.1016/j.fsc.2023.12.002
1064-7406/24/© 2023 Elsevier Inc. All rights reserved.

sensitive tissue, supports eyeglasses and face-masks, normalizes breathing by directing airflow through nostrils and away from the patient's eyes and eyeglasses, and in some cases normalizes speech. There are several methods of retaining a nasal prosthesis. The best retention method must be determined for each patient based on their anatomy, systemic health, lifestyle, and treatment goals. Creating a surgical defect that allows for ideal prosthetic design requires a team approach between the surgeon, maxillofacial prosthodontist, and anaplastologist. Additionally, a nasal prosthesis might be considered as a temporary treatment option while a patient awaits surgery.[1,8]

The journey to a finished nasal prosthesis involves 3 phases of patient care; the surgical and healing phase, possible interim prosthesis phase, and finally fabrication of the definitive prosthesis.[1,2] Typically, at least 6 weeks of healing is required before prosthesis fabrication can begin. While many traditional fine art methods and dental materials are employed in the design and fabrication of nasal prostheses, digital technology is streamlining the workflow for prosthetic rehabilitation.

## HISTORY OF FACIAL PROSTHESES

Facial prostheses were first documented in the sixteenth century by French surgeon Ambroise Paré, who is considered the founder of maxillofacial prosthetics. He is credited with the fabrication of the first nasal prosthesis made of gold, silver, and "papier mâché." A string attached to the prosthesis was tied around the head for retention. During this time, most of the prostheses were made of a combination of gold, silver, or ivory which made the prosthesis stiff and heavy. It was not until the 19th century that the materials for facial prostheses improved with the use of vulcanite, which was lighter and more comfortable for patients.[9]

Toward the end of the 19th century, Claude Martin introduced the combination of surgery and prostheses to restore defects.[10] He fabricated nasal prosthesis from translucent ceramics. Karl Henning in Austria was credited with the making of a facial prosthesis with an impression. The impression was poured in plaster with the mockup of the prosthesis being made in wax on the plaster mold. The lost-wax casting method was used to melt the wax with gelatin and glycerin paste poured into the mold with vulcanite or rubber. The prosthesis was then glued with some mastic solubilized in ether which was the most aesthetic and comfortable prosthetic fabricated at the time. This method allowed a closer representation to human tissue than previous attempts.[9]

With World War I and the resulting disfigurement, the American sculptor Anna Coleman Ladd made facial masks for soldiers with injured faces. She, along with French sculptor Jane Poupelet, worked with the American Red Cross to operate workshops for the fabrication of these masks.[9,11-15] The second half of the 20th century was marked with great improvement in the materials for facial prostheses. The development of silicone evolving into the Silastic Medical silicone elastomers allowed doctors to have medical grade silicones for facial prostheses for patients. It is still used today for facial prostheses. The work of Per-Ingvar Branemark and Tomas Albrektsson on the osseointegration of craniofacial implants paved the way for implant-retained facial prostheses. In the late seventies, Anders Tjellstrôm was the first to treat a patient with an implant-retained auricular prosthesis.[9,16-19]

## SURGICAL CONSIDERATIONS FOR TUMOR-RELATED DEFECTS OF THE NASAL COMPLEX

The most common causes of partial and total rhinectomies are squamous cell carcinomas (**Fig. 1**) and basal cell carcinomas.[5] Nasal reconstruction following removal of these tumors presents surgical and prosthetic challenges.[4] Surgical limitations include the experience of the reconstructive surgeon, as well as tissue availability and tissue health. Radiated tissue with compromised vasculature and fibrosis is particularly challenging.[1,20] Surgical reconstructive options may be further limited by the health of the patient, the need to monitor the area for recurrence, and individual patient desires to avoid additional surgery.[1] As a general rule, partial nasal defects are better served with surgical reconstruction and total nasal defects are better served with prosthetic reconstruction.[2] When possible, many patients prefer surgical reconstruction in order to avoid placing and removing a prosthesis daily.

Partial rhinectomies resulting in smaller defects can often be reconstructed prosthetically (**Fig. 2**) or surgically with great success. However, with a total nasal defect, it is often difficult to create a symmetric and esthetically pleasing result with surgical reconstruction if significant anatomic structures are removed due to the tumor.[1,2] In patients with aggressive tumors likely to recur, surgeons may prefer to have the patient wear a prosthesis instead of pursuing surgical reconstruction, so that they can monitor the surgical site closely. An interim prosthesis can be useful if a patient desires future surgical reconstruction.[8]

When the decision is made to pursue prosthetic rehabilitation, consideration should be paid to tissue quality, soft tissue mobility near the area of the

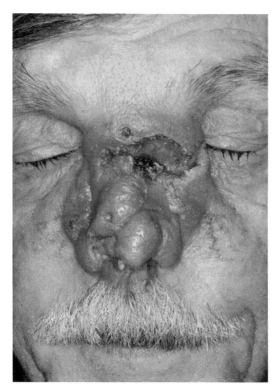

**Fig. 1.** Squamous cell carcinoma.

prosthetic margins, and possible retention options, as these factors will influence overall success and patient acceptance. In addition, careful surgical preparation of the defect greatly influences the success of the prosthesis. Surgical procedures, such as skin grafting, that reduce distortion to neighboring facial hard and soft tissues can enhance the prognosis of the prosthetic rehabilitation.[1,2] For example, if the upper lip is pulled posteriorly and superiorly during surgical closure, it will inhibit the ability to create a prosthesis with normal contours (**Fig. 3**). A retracted lip makes it difficult to conceal the lower margin of the prosthesis and can draw unwanted attention to the area. Creating a skin-lined defect is desirable in nasal defects, as unlined defects can compromise retention of the prosthesis due to delicate friable tissues, excess mucus production and drainage, and insufficient surface area for adhesive retention.[1,2] When the floor of the nasal defect is lined with a split thickness skin graft, the area can be used for excellent support of the nasal prosthesis and possible anatomic retention.

A treatment planning discussion between the surgeon and maxillofacial prosthodontist prior to surgery is crucial, as the removal of some tissues that are not affected by tumor is critical to ideal prosthetic rehabilitation (**Figs. 4** and **5**). Nasal ala

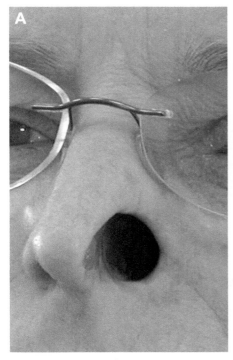
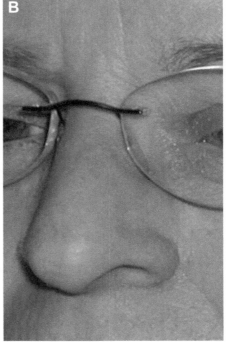

**Fig. 2.** (*A, B*): Partial nasal prosthesis.

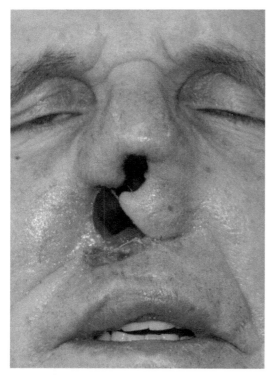

**Fig. 3.** Defect where tissue was left that prevents ideal prosthesis: bulky nasal bridge and retracted upper lip.

patient's original nasal form. Prosthetic rehabilitation for these patients requires esthetic compromises that can affect patient satisfaction. Removing otherwise-healthy nasal bones and septum can be advantageous in some instances.[1] When nasal bones and nasal bridge anatomy are retained on a partial rhinectomy patient, it is important that the soft tissues overlying these structures be as thin as possible. When the prosthesis is overcontoured over a bulky nasal bridge, the proportions of the prosthetic design can result in a restoration that is too large for the patient's facial structure. Designing a prosthetic margin over a bulky nasal bridge can also result in areas of silicone that are too thin and prone to tearing.[1] However, the decision to leave some anatomic landmarks to anchor or even retain a nasal prosthesis can be beneficial. In some cases, remnant nasal bridge and lateral sidewall structures create an anatomic undercut that can be utilized to engage a self-retained prosthesis. The nasal bridge can also provide good support for eyeglasses, which can help retain and disguise the prosthesis. Determining the ideal reconstructed nasal defect for each patient should involve collaboration between the surgeon, maxillofacial prosthodontist, anaplastologist, and other members of the healthcare team.

## METHODS OF PROSTHESIS RETENTION

Nasal prostheses can be designed to be held in place by several methods, including mechanical-retention by engaging anatomic undercuts (**Fig. 6**); adhesive-retention using various liquid adhesives or tape (**Fig. 7**); implant-retention utilizing

and nasal tip remnants often drift laterally and inferiorly when untethered from structural elements of the nose that are removed during rhinectomy like the septum and columella. This results in nasal structures that are positioned outside of the

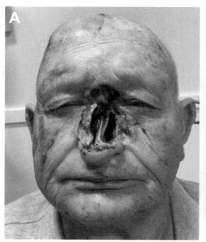
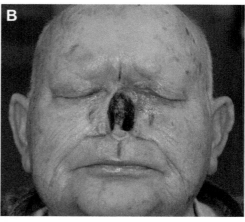

**Fig. 4.** (*A, B*): Excess tissue intentionally removed to create a defect that will allow good prosthetic outcome-requires pre-surgical collaboration.

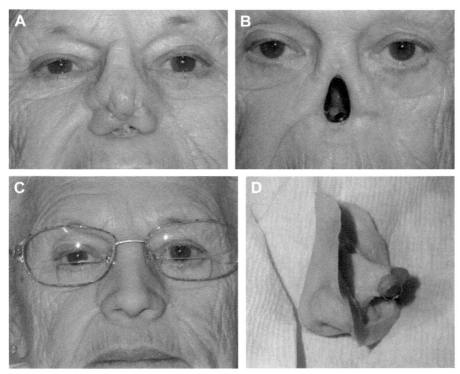

**Fig. 5.** (*A–D*): Excess tissue intentionally removed to create a defect that will allow good prosthetic outcome and breathing-requires pre-surgical collaboration. Magnet-retained prosthesis.

magnets (**Fig. 8**) or bar-and-clip structures (**Fig. 9**); or hybrid combinations of the earlier-mentioned methods. Each retention method has benefits and drawbacks and the best solution for each patient must be carefully assessed. When a self-retaining nasal prosthesis can be fabricated, this is often a highly successful and satisfactory solution. Self-retaining prostheses often include a nasal stent element, which not only holds the entire prosthesis in place, but also greatly improves breathing. However, these designs can be difficult for the maxillofacial prosthodontist and/or anaplastologist to perfect. Adhesive use is a common solution, particularly for cancer patients, but requires a considerable amount of work by the patient to apply and remove the adhesive on a daily basis. Careful cleaning of adhesive is required to avoid tearing the prosthesis or expediting silicone and color breakdown. The use of adhesives generally decreases the lifespan of the prosthesis. Implant-retained prostheses can provide improved patient satisfaction.[21,22] This type of prosthesis is easier for the patient to place and remove and often provides more reliable retention. However, not all patients are candidates for implant-retained prostheses. Patients with radiation to the site or poor systemic health may

not be candidates for implant surgery. Patients who will not be compliant with diligent implant and tissue hygiene are likewise not good candidates for implant placement. Additionally, some patients may opt for fewer surgical procedures and therefore prefer rehabilitation with an adhesive-retained prosthesis. Hybrid retention options may be advantageous by minimizing the amount of glue necessary for successful retention and avoiding the application of adhesive on the silicone edges of the prosthesis, instead relying on an adhered acrylic plate which uses magnets to engage the silicone prosthesis.

## CRANIOFACIAL IMPLANTS

Craniofacial implants employ the same design and principles of dental implants commonly used in the alveolar ridges of the maxilla and mandible. The reported success of craniofacial implants ranges widely. Studies have demonstrated implant survival rates of 93% to 100% for auricular implant, 83% to 93% for nasal implants, and 77% to 88% for orbital implants.[23–25] While some of these success rates are lower than those reported for intraoral dental implants, craniofacial implants can greatly improve retention of nasal prosthesis and

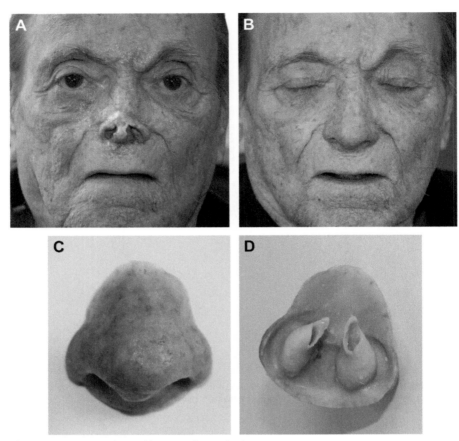

**Fig. 6.** (*A–D*): Anatomy-retained or self-retained prosthesis.

overall patient acceptance.[21,22,26] Implants should ideally be planned on a computed tomography (CT) or cone beam computed tomography (CBCT) scan with the maxillofacial prosthodontist prior to placement. Implants are placed with the prosthesis in mind to allow proper prosthesis contour and design.

Placing implants in areas with friable tissue can lead to soft tissue complications. When the anterior nasal floor is lined with a skin graft, it is a good site for implant placement. Traditionally, the best sites for placement of osseointegrated craniofacial implants are the floor of the nose and the glabella with the floor of the nose having a higher success rate. Nasal bones do not provide sufficient bone for implant placement. Therefore, if implants are planned in the glabella, the nasal bones should be removed. Implants in the nasal region have been shown to have survival rates ranging from 87.8% to 92.5%,[23–25] with radiation being a significant risk for implant loss.[27,28] More recent reports of using zygomatic implants to retain nasal prostheses have been published with promising success rates.[29] Zygomatic implants

offer several advantages. They are more likely to be out of the field of radiation and they gain more stability than traditional craniofacial implants because they pass through 3 to 4 layers of cortical bone. However, the correct placement of zygomatic implants is technique sensitive and requires planning (**Fig. 10**).[30,31]

If implants are deemed appropriate, they are placed in the chosen bony site and covered with tissue for 3 to 6 months to allow for osseointegration. During this period, an interim adhesive-retained prosthesis can be worn. Following appropriate time for osseointegration, the implants are uncovered and engaged with components used to retain the prosthesis. Typically, craniofacial implants are restored with custom bars using clips for retention or with magnets. The magnets are a popular option for facial prostheses due to easier fabrication and maintenance. The use of implant components and the elimination of adhesive allows the patient to place and remove the prosthesis with ease. Eliminating adhesive also extends the lifespan of the prosthesis, as daily cleaning of adhesive makes the silicone edges more prone to tearing.

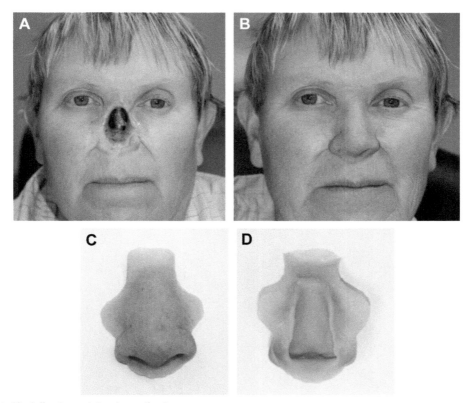

**Fig. 7.** (A–D): Adhesive-retained prosthesis.

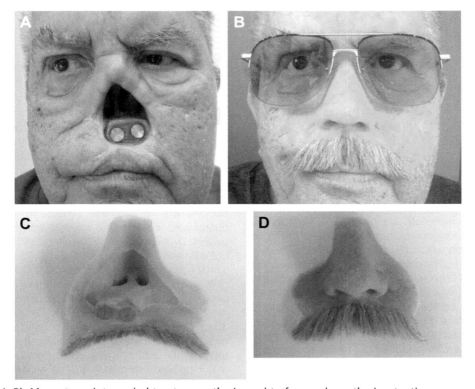

**Fig. 8.** (A–D): Magnets on intraoral obturator prosthesis used to for nasal prosthesis retention.

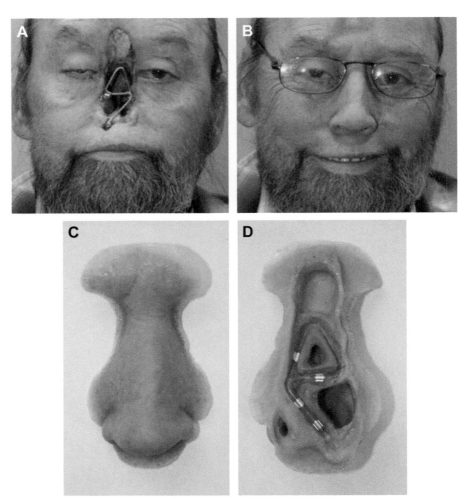

**Fig. 9.** (*A–D*): Implant-retained prosthesis utilizing an implant bar.

## PROSTHETIC FABRICATION, MATERIALS, AND TECHNIQUES

The fabrication of a nasal prosthesis requires multiple appointments following appropriate skin healing from surgery. The first visit typically involves an impression of the midface using traditional dental impression materials. Dental stone is cast in the impression, creating an accurate model of the nasal defect, upon which the prosthesis is designed in wax (**Fig. 11**). The patient then returns for a second appointment to try on the wax prosthesis. Wax is used because it can be easily modified and allows the design of the prosthesis to be changed and approved by the patient. This wax pattern is finalized, textured, and then invested in a stone mold.[32] The wax is melted out of the stone mold, leaving the negative shape of the desired prosthesis. During these appointments, color matching of the patient's pertinent anatomy takes place.

Silicone is mixed and then processed into this mold, and following silicone setting, the silicone prosthesis is recovered from the mold. Silicone can be intrinsically or extrinsically stained by the maxillofacial prosthodontist or anaplastologist (**Fig. 12**). The patient comes back for a subsequent appointment where the prosthesis is further customized with extrinsic staining and given to the patient. Digital technology can simplify this process, but still needs improvement (**Fig. 13**). Three dimensional facial scans, whether from a CT/CBCT scan or from a facial scanner, can be made of a patient's pre-op nasal contour and virtually sculpted, if the tumor distorts the shape of the nose. This can then be 3D printed, eliminating the need for hand sculpting a nasal wax pattern and can closely match the contours of the patient's pre-op nasal shape. Color matching has been digitally advanced with colorimeters like Spectromatch (Spectromatch Ltd, 27A

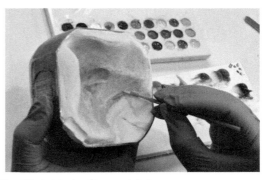

Fig. 12. Intrinsic silicone staining.

Belvedere, Lansdown Road, Bath, BA1 5HR, UK) for base shade selection.

At the prosthesis delivery appointment, time is spent educating the patient on the correct care and maintenance of their prosthesis, including donning and doffing instructions, cleaning protocols, and potential complications. The patient is then seen for regular follow up to ensure the safe and effective use of the prosthesis.

## COMPLICATIONS

Prosthetic complications are often related to issues with retention. When adhesive is used, determining the necessary type, distribution, and amount of adhesive to use for each individual takes some experimentation and trial and error. The presence of moisture from nasal drainage and condensation from air movement through the nasal prosthesis as well as constant midfacial muscle movement during speech and mastication create an environment that can be difficult for adhesives to overcome. Adhesive-retained nasal prostheses are typically remade every 1 to 2 years, due to silicone tearing or discoloration.[2] The frequency of remakes depends on the patient's hygiene, skin type, lifestyle, environment, and sun exposure.

Careful management of nasal prosthetic devices is also required in order to ensure the comfort and health of soft tissues in contact with the device. Modifications may be required to the tissue fitting surface of a nasal prosthesis if contact between the prosthesis and delicate tissues results in discomfort, pressure points, tissue breakdown, or irritation that causes excess nasal drainage. These issues may arise particularly with prostheses using anatomic retention and/or nasal stents, especially in defects not lined with skin grafts. The growth of microorganisms on the silicone surface is also sometimes seen with nasal prostheses. Microbial growth on a prosthesis can cause discoloration and possible tissue health concerns.

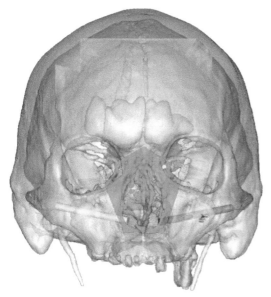

Fig. 10. Virtual surgical planning for rhinectomy and zygomatic implants.

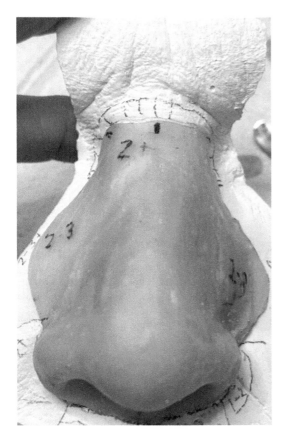

Fig. 11. Wax up of nasal prosthesis.

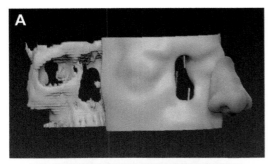

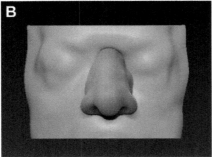

**Fig. 13.** (*A, B*): Digital design.

When microbial growth is present on a prosthesis, more frequent follow-up visits and replacement prostheses may be required.

For patients with implant-retained prostheses, the most common complications involve soft tissue reaction, most often due to lapses in hygiene.[33] Implant infection, implant failure, or implants placed in an unusable position are other possible complications. Implant components can break, lose retention, or detach from the prosthesis, so regular follow up visits are important.

Unsuccessful nasal prosthetic restoration can result from poorly designed prostheses, compromised surgical site preparation, improper implant placement, failed retention with adhesives, or patient non-compliance with care and maintenance of the device. All of these complications can be prevented or managed with good coordination and communication between patients and their surgeons, maxillofacial prosthodontists, anaplastologists, and other members of their healthcare team.

## CLINICS CARE POINTS

- Proper patient selection and a skilled surgeon are critical for successful surgical reconstruction of nasal defects. A nasal prosthesis can restore normal nasal contours, function, and esthetics if a defect is properly prepared during tumor removal.

- The promising use of zygomatic implants may result in higher implant success rates even in patients who must undergo adjuvant radiation therapy. Further studies are needed.

- The most common complication with implant-retained prostheses are soft tissue reactions. Patients who are noncompliant or unable to perform diligent hygiene may not be good candidates for craniofacial implants.

- Digital technology is improving the workflow for fabricating prostheses and skin shade matching.

- A team approach is required from the beginning of treatment for patients who will undergo a rhinectomy and subsequent prosthetic reconstruction. The maxillofacial prosthodontist and/or anaplastologist should see the patient prior to tumor resection, collaborate with the surgeon to determine if any otherwise-healthy tissues should be removed along with the tumor, and aid in prosthetically driven implant planning.

## ACKNOWLEDGMENTS

The authors would like to thank 3D Systems for providing anatomic modeling and zygomatic implant virtual planning. The authors would also like to thank Julie Brown, renowned certified anaplastologist, for her expertise and use of her images. She continually inspires us daily in the fabrication of facial prostheses.

## DISCLOSURE

There are no financial disclosures or conflicts of interest.

## REFERENCES

1. Beumer J III, Marunick MT, Espositio SJ. Maxillofacial rehabilitation: Prosthodontic and surgical management of cancer-related, Acquired, and congenital defects of the head and neck. 3rd edition. Hanover Park: Quintessence; 2011. p. 255–313.
2. Davis B, Reisberg DJ, Kirtane MV and de Souza CE. Prosthetic Rehabilitation: Intraoral and Extraoral Prostheses in Head and Neck Surgery, Otolaryngology-Head and Neck Surgery Series 2013, Thieme Medical and Scientific Publishers; Noida (India)Noida, India, 366–387.
3. Gormley M, Creaney G, Schache A, et al. Reviewing the epidemiology of head and neck cancer: definitions, trends and risk factors. Br Dent J 2022; 233(9):780–6.
4. Menick FJ. Nasal reconstruction. Plast Reconstr Surg 2010;125(4):138e–50e.

5. Plath M, Thielen HM, Baumann I, et al. Tumor Control and Quality of Life in Skin Cancer Patients With Extensive Multilayered Nasal Defects. Clin Exp Otorhinolaryngol 2020;13(2):164–72.

6. Malard O, Lanhouet J, Michel G, et al. Full-thickness nasal defect: place of prosthetic reconstruction. Eur Ann Otorhinolaryngol Head Neck Dis 2015;132(2):85–9.

7. Becker C, Becker AM, Pfeiffer J. Health-related quality of life in patients with nasal prosthesis. J Cranio-Maxillo-Fac Surg 2016;44(1):75–9.

8. Rosen EB, Golden M, Huryn JM. Fabrication of a provisional nasal prosthesis. J Prosthet Dent 2014; 112(5):1308–10.

9. Destruhaut F, Caire JM, Dubuc A, et al. Evolution of facial prosthetics: Conceptual history and biotechnological perspectives. Int J Maxillofac Prosthetics 2019;4:2–8.

10. Martin C. De la prothèse immédiate à la résection des maxillaires. Paris: éditions Masson Ed; 1889.

11. Destruhaut F, Esclassan R, ToulouseE Vigarios E, et al. A history of prosthetic skin from the First World War until now. Actes, French Society for the History of Dental Art 2012;17:55–8.

12. Sigaux N, Amiel M, Piotrovitch d'Orlik S, et al. Albéric Pont, la grande guerre et les gueules cassées (Alberic Pont, the great war and the "broken faces"). Ann Chir Plast Esthet 2017;62:601–8.

13. Williams M, Tong DC, Ansell M. Plates for masking facial wounds. J Roy Army Med Corps 2014;160:51–3.

14. Wood FD. Masks for Facial Wounds. Lancet 1917; 189:949–51.

15. Baron P, Dussourt E. Anna Coleman Ladd (1878-1938), workshop designer of Studio for Portrait Masks in Paris. Cah Prot 2018 2018;182:32–51.

16. Colas A, Curtis J. silicone biomaterials: History and chemistry. Biomaterials science: An introduction to materials in medicine 2004; 2:80-85.

17. Andres CJ, Haug SP, Munoz CA, et al. Effects of environmental factors on maxillofacial elastomers: Part I-Literature review. J Prosthetic Dent 1992;68:327–30.

18. Tjellstrom A, Lindstrom J, Nylen O, et al. The bone-ancholored auricular episthesis. Laryngoscope 1981;91:811–5.

19. Federspil PA. Implant-retained craniofacial prostheses for facial defects. GMS Curr Top Otorhinolaryngol, Head Neck Surg 2009;8:03.

20. Straub JM, New J, Hamilton CD, et al. Radiation-induced fibrosis: mechanisms and implications for therapy. J Cancer Res Clin Oncol 2015;141(11):1985–94.

21. Chang TL, Garrett N, Roumanas E, et al. Treatment satisfaction with facial prostheses. J Prosthet Dent 2005;94(3):275–80.

22. Nemli SK, Aydin C, Yilmaz H, et al. Quality of life of patients with implant-retained maxillofacial prostheses: a prospective and retrospective study. J Prosthet Dent 2013;109(1):44–52.

23. Alberga J, Eggels I, Visser A, et al. Outcome of implants placed to retain craniofacial prostheses - A retrospective cohort study with a follow-up of up to 30 years. Clin Implant Dent Relat Res 2022;24(5):643–54.

24. Chrcanovic BR, Nilsson J, Thor A. Survival and complications of implants to support craniofacial prosthesis: A systematic review. J Cranio-Maxillo-Fac Surg 2016;44(10):1536–52.

25. Curi MM, Oliveira MF, Molina G, et al. Extraoral implants in the rehabilitation of craniofacial defects: implant and prosthesis survival rates and peri-implant soft tissue evaluation. J Oral Maxillofac Surg 2012;70(7):1551–7.

26. Rosen EB, Ahmed ZU, Huryn JM, et al. Prosthetic rehabilitation of the geriatric oncologic rhinectomy patient utilizing a craniofacial implant-retained nasal prosthesis. Clin Case Rep 2019;8(2):278–82.

27. Granström G, Tjellström A, Brånemark PI, et al. Bone-anchored reconstruction of the irradiated head and neck cancer patient. Otolaryngol Head Neck Surg 1993;108(4):334–43.

28. Chrcanovic BR, Albrektsson T, Wennerberg A. Dental implants in irradiated versus nonirradiated patients: A meta-analysis. Head Neck 2016;38(3): 448–81.

29. Scott N, Kittur MA, Evans PL, et al. The use of zygomatic implants for the retention of nasal prosthesis following rhinectomy: the Morriston experience. Int J Oral Maxillofac Surg 2016;45(8):1044–8.

30. Rosenstein J, Dym H. Zygomatic Implants: A Solution for the Atrophic Maxilla: 2021 Update. Dent Clin North Am 2021;65(1):229–39.

31. Aparicio C, Manresa C, Francisco K, et al. Zygomatic implants: indications, techniques and outcomes, and the zygomatic success code. Periodontol 2000 2014; 66(1):41–58.

32. Acharya V, Montgomery PC. A technique to orient a stone cast in the fabrication of a nasal prosthesis. J Prosthet Dent 2014;112(3):692–4.

33. Karakoca S, Aydin C, Yilmaz H, et al. Survival rates and periimplant soft tissue evaluation of extraoral implants over a mean follow-up period of three years. J Prosthet Dent 2008;100(6):458–64.

# *Moving?*

## *Make sure your subscription moves with you!*

To notify us of your new address, find your **Clinics Account Number** (located on your mailing label above your name), and contact customer service at:

**Email: journalscustomerservice-usa@elsevier.com**

**800-654-2452** (subscribers in the U.S. & Canada)
**314-447-8871** (subscribers outside of the U.S. & Canada)

**Fax number: 314-447-8029**

**Elsevier Health Sciences Division
Subscription Customer Service
3251 Riverport Lane
Maryland Heights, MO 63043**

*To ensure uninterrupted delivery of your subscription, please notify us at least 4 weeks in advance of move.

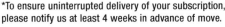

Printed and bound by CPI Group (UK) Ltd, Croydon, CR0 4YY

08/05/2025

01864724-0019